Deep IMMUNITY

Understanding Your Body's Immune System

THIRD EDITION

Anthony Godfrey B.V.Sc., D.T.V.M., Ph.D., N.D.

DEEP IMMUNITY:
Understanding Your Body's Immune System

St. Francis Herb Farm®
P.O. Box 29
Combermere, ON K0J 1L0
Canada

ISBN-13: 978-1-926676-78-4

Editors: Mark Sebanc and James Anderson (www.stoneharp.com)
Layout: James Anderson and Paul Probert
Cover Design: Word Alive Press

Printed in Canada.

Printed by Word Alive Press
131 Cordite Road, Winnipeg, MB R3W 1S1
www.wordalivepress.ca

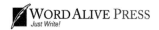

WORD ALIVE PRESS
Just Write!

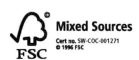

Mixed Sources
Cert no. SW-COC-001271
© 1996 FSC

FSC

to

SARAH, ERIN,
CLARA and GLADYS

*my teachers, my inspiration
and my support.*

ACKNOWLEDGEMENTS

I cannot count and certainly cannot name the tens of thousands of students and thousands of clients who have inspired me to seek a greater understanding of the process of healing. These beloved people, and a host of authors whose books have opened new levels of perspective, context and wisdom for me, have been and continue to be among my greatest teachers. I am also continually taught about myself, about life, and about the healing journey by healing plants, by all aspects of nature, and by the Creator of All. I extend my heartfelt thanks to them all.

I am ever inspired by my two grown daughters, whose efforts to understand the meaning of life and participate fully in it make me feel like a beginner. Their goodness, wisdom and maturity are a constant inspiration to me, and my life would be empty without them.

My mother Gladys has always been my strongest and most enthusiastic supporter. At nearly 95 years of age, she has great vitality, is interested in all facets of life, and is an inspiration to all who have the privilege to know her. I am deeply blessed to have her as a close friend and advisor.

I especially want to thank my wife Sarah, who in addition to running our home and caring for our family, manages my clinical practice, types my manuscripts, and is my bridge to the mysterious world of computers and electronic communication. Working together on so many levels brings us closer, and I am indeed fortunate to have such a loving and accomplished life partner. I cannot find the words to describe the depth of my appreciation and love for her. It's a feeling—it's in my heart.

Lastly, I want to thank Monique and Jeremy of St. Francis Herb Farm for their enduring friendship and their wonderful herbal remedies. My editors, Mark Sebanc and Jim Anderson, authors of *The Stoneholding*, have made the work a pleasure, always maintaining optimism, sensitivity, and good humour. Thank you!

ANTHONY GODFREY

Toronto, Canada

SEPTEMBER 2005

TABLE OF CONTENTS

CHAPTER ONE
An Introduction to Deep Immunity

THE NATURE OF IMMUNITY

Right relationships are the basis of immunity. It's about balance—balance within ourselves, with our environment, and with the whole universe. It's not about isolation, about making ourselves invulnerable to attack. Rather, it is a matter of living in harmony with everything around us. As we express our true selves in relationship to the world around us, we help create harmony rather than warfare. In cooperation with the created order around us, we enter into communion with our world. The key to communion, this harmony of being, is that each one of us in the great chain of being lives true to his nature—that is, with integrity.

These relationships work best when each of us remains focused on expressing his own deepest identity as a created being and does so in the knowledge that his existence is not an accident, but that every thing has a rightful place in the universe. With this self-awareness comes respect for the other creatures in the environment and out of this grows a harmonious synergy of life.

But this is not a perfect world, or, more specifically, we humans are not perfect. There is much disharmony. In recent times, the expression of identity and the definition of boundaries have become more aggressive, responding to *attack* with *counter-attack*. The modern language of immunity is militaristic: it speaks of immunity to *attack* by micro-organisms, about mounting a *defence* or a *counter-attack*. While it is almost impossible—even in this book—to avoid using this language, it does not capture the real power of immunity. The real power of immunity comes from being true to ourselves—each of us to our own identity. As we express ourselves with integrity, we enter into a respectful, cooperative, and harmonious relationship with all the inhabitants of the world around us.

Learning to Listen

Good health is one of the most highly valued of life's attributes, but for most of us it is elusive. The symptoms of ill-health are a language that the body, the mind, and the spirit speak to us to indicate that something in our life is out of balance. When we desire to live in integrity and in harmony with ourselves and our environment, we learn to interpret the language of ill-health. Small symptoms, maybe just an awareness that something is not quite right, attract our attention and help us to recognize the disharmony within ourselves. With this recognition, we can respond in a positive way to restore the balance. As we begin to trust our response to the symptoms of ill-health, we feel a growing sense of confidence and actually begin to feel alive in a way we could not before.

Instead of reacting in fear and in uncertainty, resigning ourselves to the condition of ill health, we can follow the path to wellness and wholeness of being.

Fear isolates. When we feel isolated, we lose our sense of self and our sense of relatedness to the world around us. No longer knowing our place in the world, we experience a loss of equilibrium. There's no need to fear ill-health. Ill-health is an indication that we are out of balance—that we are not living true to ourselves and are also out of harmony with our environment and the creatures in it. If we react to ill-health in fear, then we depress our immune response, but if our response is to acknowledge that we are part of a greater whole and that our symptoms indicate that we are out of harmony with ourselves and that greater whole, then our immune system becomes stronger and we begin to return to health.

Occasionally we meet a person who has lost the will to live. This situation is dire because we know that immunity and the ability to restore health depend on a positive use of one's will. A person can only lose the will to live when he has lost his sense of identity. If he rediscovers the sense of self, then he reclaims his will, the will to live fully and even to live happily a death that is inevitable. Life is an expression of our ability to respond, to be responsive, responsible—not in the sense of being a good person fulfilling all of our commitments, but inwardly always holding in our hearts the vision of what we believe we can become and those things that we believe it is our gift to be a part of, to foster, and to bring into being.

The Meaning of Self and Non-Self

Self and non-self—these are distinctions we can make between that which is a part of me or that which I am and that which lies beyond or outside of me. These terms speak not simply about our physical being, but, in a more complete sense, about our totality as a physical and psycho-spiritual being. We must each determine this difference between self and non-self.

This determination of self and non-self will allow us to come into possession of our true self and all that we are. When we come to this self-possession and can express our sense of self clearly and with integrity, others will be apt to perceive this expression of self in a vivid and immediate, almost palpable, way. This has been described as a "presence" of the person or the manifestation of a person's spiritual identity. The more self-possessed we are and the more connected we are to our identity, the greater will be this perceived presence. This is merely an indication that we have taken our proper place in the world around us, enabling ourselves to build the best immune system possible. This knowledge of self and its expression manifests a perfect immunity—I know who I am and who I am not, what I am and what I am not.

Thus we can create better relationships, because, when others see who we are and that we are secure and at peace in our existence, they also feel secure and are inspired to look to their own deeper needs, issues, and identity. This happens in all relationships, not just with our fellow human beings, but with all of creation.

Determining Physical Boundaries

Let us look now at immunity on the physical level. Awareness of ourselves and of our environment is the first criterion for good immunity. How does our body know what is happening to it and when it might be compromised? Our bodies are vigilant. People who are very unaware of their bodies often get more seriously sick than those who are vigilant, or their symptoms become more advanced before they seek help. Vigilance does not mean worrying, being a hypochondriac or constantly going for check-ups—it means being aware of subtle disturbances to our peace and the sense of wellbeing that we should feel. What should follow next is an appropriate response—a slight course correction, if you like, to bring us back into balance.

Our skin is our major interface with the outside world. It can tell us if we are getting too cold or too hot, or whether we are wet and likely to get chilled and catch a cold as a result of the wind blowing on us. An appropriate response is to wrap up warmly or remove some clothes, to dry off, or protect ourselves from the wind and perhaps have a warm drink or warm soup. Such actions are common sense. They are the first use of immune sense.

Establishing Psycho-Spiritual Boundaries

Immunity, based upon the awareness of our own self identity, is important on another level. All of us at times are aware that we are under psychological or spiritual attack—that someone is projecting negativity at us. In arguments we can feel the angry words tearing into us or feel the penetration of hatred or jealousy or envy from another's eyes. Conversely, just as people can penetrate our personal space with their consciousness and deposit negative energy there, they can also, if we allow them, gain entry and steal a part of our energy or our consciousness. I am sure many of us have experienced this too, that some people leave us feeling uncharacteristically depleted, exhausted or emotional—perhaps sad, guilty or lacking in self-esteem.

How then do we protect ourselves from these influences? This is a matter of immunity also. In fact, through a strong sense of self, the boundaries of our consciousness are strengthened. We become more aware of negativity approaching us and can refuse entry to it more successfully. If there has been some violation or if we feel the negativity still sticking to us, we can re-establish the boundaries of self and reclaim our peace.

In fact, psychological and spiritual violations of any kind are contrary to the basic laws of the universe. That we disobey these laws is a fundamental reason why we perceive immunity in militaristic terms. Once we strive to live true to our self-identity, in self-possession and with respect for all creation, our concept of immunity changes.   —ve

So, which works best? The fortress approach, where we cut ourselves off from the outside world and respond to attack with merciless counter-attack? Or the harmonious approach, based on +ve improved self-awareness and a fuller expression of identity and mutual respect? While some might say that ideally the harmonious approach would work best and might be willing to give it a try, I suspect that in practice most people still support the fortress approach. I hope to show in this short book that the strongest, most enduring and, thus, most successful immunity is built on cooperation and mutual respect. I will also show that as long as we perpetuate the fortress approach, our immune problems will multiply.

Joy is a word we don't hear much, but joy is what we begin to feel as we develop true immunity. It comes from being in a right relationship with everything in the world and beyond, from living a life fully expressive of our truest, deepest nature. It is a loving and respectful relationship that creates joy within us and around us.

THE PURPOSE OF THIS BOOK

Appreciation of the miraculous working of your immune system can only serve to empower you. It will give you both a greater understanding of the mechanisms of immunity and a greater ability to utilize, strengthen, balance, and direct it. Modern science is only beginning to understand how the immune system works. The detail and complexity seem endless. As one branch of science, the reductionist branch, probes deeper and deeper into smaller and smaller fragments of the mechanism, another branch, that of quantum physics, looks outward. Contemporary science and medicine have discovered that in many ways we determine our own reality, and that, in fact, we are capable of determining our very selves in every instant and that what we hold as our deepest beliefs about ourselves and our relationship to the rest of the universe determines, in a very real way, how we feel, how well we function and, as a result of this, how our immune system works.

In this book I will share an introductory understanding of both these viewpoints—one the reductionist, Cartesian or Newtonian view, the other a post-Einsteinian one. The latter blends vividly with the experiences of mystics and other deeply aware and self-aware people. In case you are not familiar with these more recent developments in our understanding, I will provide a bibliography of suggested reading at the end of the book.

I am writing this book from my perspective as a naturopathic doctor. Naturopathic doctors hold five principles which guide their practice of medicine and their relationship with their clients. The first principle, "First Do No Harm," which we share with medical doctors, is attributed to Hippocrates, one of the founding fathers of modern medicine. This is followed by the second principle, "Find and Treat The Cause." In order to discover the cause of a person's ill health, a cause which may originate at the physical level, but usually has emotional, mental, and spiritual components as well, we must come to know the whole person.

"Treat the Whole Person" is the third of our principles, meaning that we must take into account that the symptoms the person is experiencing may have their origin at a deeper level. Physical symptoms may be related to emotions, to mental stress or be a result of negative beliefs or attitudes which diminish rather than build the person up. If there is an openness, then it is important to treat the person at these deeper levels.

The process of healing is most successful when it is assisted and guided by nature. The healing power of nature—in Latin, the *Vis Medicatrix Naturae*—is a power which lies within us and all of creation. Our fourth principle is to "Employ the Healing Power of Nature." This power is found in sunshine, fresh air, pure water, earth, and the plants that grow on the earth. It can facilitate healing and move us in that direction by reminding us what it feels like to be well. I will discuss all these factors in detail below in my role as a conveyor of our fifth principle: "Doctor as Teacher."

The following sections provide an overview of the material to be discussed in this book.

The Physiological Components of the Immune System

Antibodies are the proteins that the body creates to neutralize foreign substances that compromise the health of the body. Antibodies are produced by cells called B-lymphocytes and are one of our main defences against micro-organisms. Unfortunately, we can mistakenly make antibodies to substances that are not, in and of themselves, harmful, such as cat dander, ragweed pollen, peanuts or shellfish. We will discuss antibodies as part of what is called *humoral immunity*.

Cells contribute to immunity in other ways as well. Several classes of cells can attract, consume (phagocytose), and destroy bacteria, other micro-organisms, cancer cells, and unwanted debris in the body. This is called *cellular immunity*.

Lastly, there are several classes of chemical components released by cells in an immune response which facilitate cell mobilization, cell production, antibody production, and cell movement and which potentiate the effectiveness of antibodies in their efforts to protect us.

Causes of a Compromised Immune System

The immune system has certain essential requirements during its development in infancy and childhood, which, if not met, gives us a rocky start. We humans have evolved in co-existence with the other creatures of the earth, most importantly, micro-organisms. In order to create a balanced cooperative relationship with the many species of bacteria, fungi, and other organisms that live in us and on us, we need a proper introduction to them. There are trillions of micro-organisms in each of us, and we need them as much as they need us. If we don't start our lives in a consistent environment, with healthy parents and a normal vaginal birth followed by breast-feeding, problems can arise.

The effort to separate or isolate ourselves from the environment in which these organisms live backfires. It is an example of how ignoring or trying to modify the laws of nature, within which we evolved, results in separation from the healing power of nature. Under such unnatural circumstances, the developing infant immune system can become overwhelmed. Even though it is not easy for many of us to provide a natural start for our children, it is reassuring to know that it is usually possible to correct these early problems. To get the best results, however, we must come back into harmony with nature, not move further away from her.

Restoring the Immune System

Nurturing ourselves and one another is the fastest way to recover our health and balance our immunity. Nurturing means supplying healing help, nourishment, care, concern, and listening. Listening is a vital part of nurturing. In order to contribute to healing, we must listen for signs of distress, listen to the emotions, to body language, to unspoken evidence of pain, damage, hurt, trauma—all the factors which create imbalance in us or another person. Through listening, we learn how to approach the situation in truth with a positive mental attitude and can provide elements of nurturing, be it food, a cool bath, or a herbal remedy. Thus balance begins to be restored.

The act of listening and responding compassionately and appropriately not only helps a person to come back into balance, but it gives them strength. That strength comes because of our intent to listen (without judgment) to (respond with compassion.) The strength does not come from us, but rather it flows through us. We facilitate healing by trying to come into harmony with the laws of healing and by seeking to be agents of healing by holding unconditional love for the person in need—be they ourselves or another.

Rebuilding and Maintaining an Effective Immune System

If we are well-balanced, our immunity will be strong, and we will be able to detect the beginnings of imbalance. Until we become attuned to self-balance, we may not notice anything wrong until something really serious gets our attention—a crushing headache, the inability to breathe, a pain which makes us double over— any of a whole range of physical symptoms. We should also realize we are far out of balance if we are overly emotional—fearful, anxious, vengeful, uncontrollably angry, self-destructive, or, as mentioned, resigned to self-deprecating judgement, losing ourselves and our way spiritually. With practice, however, our vigilance will pay off, and we will detect the slightest disturbance to our inner or outer balance. This developing self-awareness and our increasing (sensitivity to our environment) allow us to enter into a cooperative relationship, working with any unbalancing factor, whether from within or without.

Let us start with an example of inner imbalance. If we feel fear and are able to acknowledge it, we can then ask help from another to (alleviate that fear,) drawing on or accessing the courage that another can hold for us. In time we realize that courage also lies within us and we can learn to access it ourselves. The ability to manage our fear is already a part of our identity, and we will discuss how to make such inner transitions later.

If our (imbalance) is caused by an outer factor, our symptoms, if carefully observed, will lead us to a remedy. We are cold—but (why?) Maybe it is cold where we are, or, then again, perhaps our energy is low because we haven't eaten recently or are overtired. Maybe our circulation needs help. Appropriate actions and appropriate herbal remedies can restore balance and good health.

The Unique Contribution of Herbal Remedies

Specific Medication is the title of a book written in the late 19th century by an Eclectic Physician by the name of John Scudder. He was a leading light in herbalism's golden era and enjoyed great success because he realized that each medicinally useful plant carried specific qualities. These qualities included their physical nature, their chemical constituents, but went far beyond chemistry to address, by their essence or energetic qualities, the deeper imbalances within the person. Homeopathy, a branch of holistic medicine that developed early in the 19th century, uses only the energetic properties of plants and other substances to support healing, and Scudder was able to tie the two together—the physical and the energetic. His ability to match a healing herb to the needs of an individual and his evaluations of the specific healing qualities of plants have stood the test of time.

Traditional Chinese medical doctors also understood this balance of the physical and the energetic and developed sensitive diagnostic methods to determine which specific plants should be utilized in order to restore harmonious functioning. Although most of this work was done before the era of modern scientific investigation, their intuitive understanding of the healing qualities of plants is being borne out by modern research.

Finding the Best Herbal Immune Product

No two people are alike. No two cases of a disease are alike. Even in two people with the same diagnosis, disease does not develop, nor will it progress, in the same way. This means the physician must treat each person as a unique case. We must each look at ourselves in the same way. We have the freedom and the responsibility to choose the specific path of healing which seems to suit our own situation best. In order to do this, we may need the help of a skilled diagnostician and a skilled herbalist. If we are encouraged to cooperate fully in the history-taking—the listening—and feel good about the diagnosis and the plan of treatment, then we should arrive at the most appropriate approach for our unique situation.

The skilled herbalist will then combine the appropriate herbs to make your first remedy. As you begin to recover, this remedy may be modified or other remedies added, to support you on your healing journey.

Quality herbs are essential to this process. You may find a skilled diagnostician, a brilliant compounder, but if the herbs themselves lack vitality or have been poorly stored and perhaps damaged by mould, radiation or contamination, their full potential to heal will not be available to you.

When the Immune System Is Most in Need of Support

Stress of any kind will weaken our immune systems. Stress, or more correctly, the nature of our response to challenges which tend to disturb or unbalance us, can come in many forms. Some of us, for example, are susceptible to the challenges of extreme weather conditions. For others, the responsibilities of being a parent, a teacher, a nurse or a doctor, where people are dependent on you and draw on you, may be very stressful. For yet others, life itself and the attempt to make good decisions can cause anxiety and worry, which in turn cause an increase in adrenaline levels, a physiological response which we know depresses the immune system.

Physical challenges such as weather, lack of sleep, inadequate nutrition, lack of exercise and limited access to the healing power of the natural environment will create a need for immune support.

To some extent, we can offset these physical effects by connecting to our inner sense of self and rebuilding our presence from within, thereby becoming recollected and strengthening our self-possession. Psycho-spiritual attacks can bring us down if we are not able to protect ourselves, but the most devastating influence of all is negative self-talk. When we allow ourselves to embrace negative beliefs about ourselves, when we fall into despair and lack of self-esteem and become resigned to these judgements about ourselves—in other words, when we lose our identity—that is when our immune system is most in need of support.

CHAPTER TWO
How the Immune System Works

THE HUMAN IMMUNE SYSTEM

White blood cells, found both in our blood and also in many other parts of our body, are the most important components of the immune system.

Some white blood cells have as their major responsibility the recognition and destruction of pathogenic micro-organisms, such as bacteria, and abnormal cells, such as cancer cells. These cells fall into special groups. There are cells in the bloodstream called neutrophils or "polys" (polymorphonuclear leucocytes), which are a bit like "pac-men" and devour micro-organisms in the blood. Cells in the tissues are sometimes quite mobile and, in fact, use the bloodstream as a transit system to get where they are needed. Cells called monocytes, when we find them in the blood, and macrophages (big eaters), when we find them in the tissues, are major consumers of products of inflammation—bacteria, debris, and dead cells. Another major tissue cell is called a histiocyte (which means tissue cell), and every kind of tissue has its own variety. Most of these histiocyctes are fixed in the tissues and together make up a network of defensive cells called the reticulo-endothelial system. Other white blood cells called lymphocytes have, as their major responsibility, the recognition of foreign materials in the body called antigens and the manufacture of specific antibodies to those antigens. In the inventory of the body, antibodies are available to every known substance. A lymphocyte is type-specific to the kind of antibody it creates. When it encounters an antigen, a lymphocyte springs into action and starts making an antigen-specific antibody. Having once produced some antibody for a certain antigen, this specific cell, now called a B-lymphocyte, can respond much more quickly to subsequent encounters with that same antigen.

The cells of the immune system constitute what we call the *cellular immune system*. The antibodies and antibody recognition and response mechanisms are known as the *humoral immune system*. In addition to these two major divisions, there are untold numbers of regulating mechanisms at work in different tissues and under different circumstances—these are controlled by chemical mediators.

For those who wish to learn more on the subject, a more detailed and precise description of the immune system is presented in the following three sections.

The Principal Types of Human Immunity

Innate immunity: This immunity is comprised of a series of standard mechanisms, common to all healthy people, the effectiveness of which depends on the general health of the tissues. The components of innate immunity are:

- the resistance of the skin to invasion, which is a function of its tough design combined with surface antibodies and a host of protective micro-organisms that together make the skin an inhospitable resting place for pathogenic organisms.

- destruction of pathogenic organisms and some toxic substances by stomach acid and digestive enzymes.

- phagocytosis and destruction of organisms and debris by the white blood cells and macrophages in the blood and tissues.

- chemicals found in the blood which attach to foreign organisms or toxins. These are of three kinds:

  1) lysozymes, which attach to and cause the dissolution of the organisms or toxins.

  2) a class of protein called polypeptides, which can neutralize certain kinds of bacteria, mostly of the Gram negative type, e.g., coliforms like E-coli.

  3) a complex of about 20 or more proteins, which form a co-ordinated system to assist other immune functions. This is called the complement system.

Acquired immunity: Acquired or specific immunity is gradually built up in the newborn and throughout life as a result of exposure to micro-organisms and potentially antigenic molecules in our environment. This branch of immunity is much more reliant than innate immunity upon appropriate support for its development, both early in life and later.

Acquired immunity is orders of magnitude more powerful than innate immunity and can protect us from challenges that would devastate an individual not similarly prepared.

Acquired immunity is located in lymphoid tissue, which includes lymph nodes, the spleen, the Peyer's patches of the small intestinal wall, and the lymphoid cells of the bone marrow, as well as aggregations of lymphatic cells, such as tonsils and diffuse distributions of lymphocytes in connective tissue all over the body.

The action of the acquired immune system occurs through activated lymphocytes on the one hand and antibodies made by modified lymphocytes on the other.

How Acquired Immunity Is Created and Activated

Specific proteins or large polysaccharides (complex sugars) with a molecular weight above 8000 are called antigens. It is these antigenic substances that stimulate the lymphoid tissue to respond. When an antigen enters the body or comes in contact with lymphoid tissues directly under the mucosal and epithelial surfaces, such as the lining of the digestive and respiratory systems, there are two kinds of response—the cellular and the humoral responses.

The Cellular Response: In the cellular response, a particular strain of so-called T-lymphocyte will recognize the antigen and become active. There are millions of different kinds of T-lymphocytes, each pre-programmed to recognize a different antigen. The lymphocytes can be stimulated to destroy the foreign substance or organism, either by direct contact with it, or, more often, by contact with antigenic residues ejected by macrophages that have already phagocytosed, killed and broken down the foreign material. Once activated, the T-cells begin to multiply and travel throughout the body, taking up position in readiness to neutralize the foreign material wherever they encounter it.

The Humoral Response: Another type of lymphocyte called a B-lymphocyte is pre-programmed to make antibodies. Just as there are millions of kinds of T-lymphocytes, there are millions of kinds of B-lymphocytes. Each type is capable of making a particular antibody to neutralize one specific antigen. The B-lymphocytes begin to multiply in response to contact with a specific antigen or the byproducts of macrophage activity. These rapidly multiplying B-cells have to undergo one more step before they can produce antibody—they must enlarge and turn into an antibody-making plasma cell. This transition from B-cell to plasma cell is aided by signals from the T-lymphocytes that have encountered the same antigen. Antibody levels build up in the tissues and in the blood and lymphatic systems, neutralizing the antigen and forming antibody-antigen complexes. The cells continue to multiply, and the initial response may last a few days to a few weeks.

The Memory of an Acquired Immune Response

T-cells that have encountered and responded to an antigen become distributed throughout the lymphoid tissues of the body. On the next occasion of exposure to the same antigen, the T-lymphocytes will increase in number much more quickly than on the first exposure.

B-cells that have been activated by antigens turn into plasma cells for the most part, in order to produce their specific antibodies, but a small portion of the exposed B-cell population remains as lymphocytes. These cells are called memory cells, and they are distributed all over the lymphoid tissue in readiness for subsequent challenges. In both T-cells and B-cells a second response is much faster, more powerful, and longer-lasting than the first response. This is a very rudimentary description of how the human immune system works. The more research is done, the more complex the subject of immunity becomes.

THE IMMUNE SYSTEM IN ACTION

Micro-organisms such as bacteria, viruses, and moulds trigger our immune system. We are all aware that we have immune defences against these minute creatures that have the potential to cause disease in our bodies. However, people are often less aware that we also have antibodies responsive to lectins, a component of food. Which foods we have antibodies for depends on our blood type. For the majority of people, these antibodies are found in all secretions, such as saliva, digestive juices, tears, and perspiration, as well as in the blood. In addition, the immune system is able to recognize cellular debris from aging and dead cells as well as abnormal cells, such as cancer cells, which it destroys as part of the health maintenance program of the body.

If we are in contact with substances of a molecular weight below 8000, such as drugs, some chemicals, animal dander, old skin and poison ivy oil, we can still mount an immune response. The immune system binds a large protein molecule to the smaller irritating molecule, which is known as a hapten, and then antibodies are formed which can, in the future, respond to and neutralize either the specific protein or the hapten. This response is a mixed blessing in that, while it protects the body, it may also trigger inflammation and allergy.

The more balanced and strong our immune systems are and the less inflammation there is in our bodies, the less likely this negative reaction is to happen. These so-called sensitivities or allergies which we develop are not a healthy reaction and are preventable and usually correctable.

Homeostasis means the ability of the body to keep all its vital functions within normal limits. Our body temperature, for example, must be kept very close to 37° C (98.6° F), and the electrolytes (minerals) in tissues, cells, and blood must be maintained within very narrow limits. Although blood pressure, heart and respiration rate, and the frequency of urination or bowel activity may vary from moment to moment, or even day to day, these functions must remain within certain ranges for us to stay healthy. Most of these mechanisms are automatic and happen naturally without any special effort on our part. Most of the control comes from a part of the nervous system called the autonomic nervous system, meaning it is autonomous, working on its own without voluntary intervention from us. If these normal measurements and rhythms are out of range and if the necessary mechanisms are not automatically maintaining homeostasis, we have reason to suspect that something is wrong, and it usually is.

In addition to the automatic mechanisms, we have those behaviours which we perform voluntarily to stay healthy. For example, we try to warm up when we are cold by adding clothes or going to a warmer place. We eat when we are hungry. If our bowel movements are sluggish, we will add more fibre to our diets and make sure we are drinking enough water—at least we should. Vigilance concerning our body's state and its needs is very important.

Openings into the body, such as the mouth, the nose, and the genital and rectal openings are heavily guarded by the immune system. Each of these, and any other natural opening—the eyes or the openings of sweat glands, for example—have lymphatic tissue associated with them.

Take the mouth as an example. Organisms can enter the mouth and travel from the mouth down the esophagus to the stomach. On their way from lips to esophagus, bacteria have to pass over our tongue and through the pharynx. The pharynx is a passageway at the back of the mouth which is the intersection between our main food tube, the esophagus, and our air pathway. Air comes in through our nose or mouth and passes through the pharynx before descending by way of the larynx or voice box into our airways and lungs. The food path actually crosses the air path because the trachea—the main airway to the lungs—lies in front of the esophagus. So we have a complex mechanism to close the larynx while we swallow. Laughter, talking, and eating quickly as we breathe can sometimes cause us to inhale food or water by accident. At such times we cough violently to clear the airways. Coming into the pharynx near the back are two tubes to the middle ear on each side called Eustachian tubes. If they are inflamed or partially blocked, bacteria can enter and infect these tubes.

The body's major defence for all these important and vulnerable openings is to surround the area with a ring of lymphatic tissue. If you look at the back of your tongue in a mirror, you can see a lot of lumps and bumps. These are the lingual tonsils. Just beside the back of the tongue, one on either side, are two bean-shaped pharyngeal tonsils; however, these are often partially hidden by flaps of mouth skin. We have tonsils in the palate, called palatine tonsils, which, when swollen and infected, are called adenoids.

Wounds and breaks in the skin or any lining surfaces, such as mucous membranes or serous membranes, which cover respectively the insides and outsides of our internal organs, are vulnerable to attack by pathogenic, that is, disease-causing organisms. At wound sites we usually do not have specialized lymphatic tissue, but rely on our general immune response, which is activated as soon as inflammation occurs.

Unbroken skin is protection in itself, since it is quite tough, but antibodies and protective bacteria are found all over the skin, ready to protect us from the vast number of organisms we encounter every moment.

The ileocaecal valve is an example of the meeting of a dirty zone, the colon, with a clean zone, the small intestine. All intestinal contents must pass through the ileocaecal valve, where the small intestine empties into the large intestine. This valve is usually tightly closed, except when the contents of the small intestine, called chyme, are passing through. Right on the other side of the valve is the appendix. People have speculated on the origin and role of the appendix, but close examination shows it is full of lymphatic tissue—it protects us.

Lymphatic tissue is located strategically around all the natural entry points into the body. How does it work? Tonsils in the pharyngeal area are balls of lymphatic tissue into which the lining of the mouth dips quite deeply. In the case of the pharyngeal tonsils, the ones we simply call tonsils and which are surgically removed at times, the mucosa dips very deeply and forms crypts into which

bacteria and other organisms in the pharynx may fall. As these organisms set up house in the tonsillar crypts, lymphatic cells check
them out and, if they are dangerous organisms, start the process of
antibody production. So the tonsillar tissue of the pharynx and the
appendix at the ileocaecal valve are like a customs checkpoint,
sampling the organisms that travel by and taking appropriate action.

Healing is the response to any break in the skin or the mucosal
or serosal barriers. The initial response to a wound varies in intensity with the degree of trauma, but even a small cut, enough to ad-
mit some pathogenic organisms, will generate a response. Cells in
the tissues have been damaged, and among them are so-called mast
cells. When mast cells are damaged, they release histamine, a
chemical which makes the blood vessels in the immediate area
more permeable. This causes fluid and immune cells to escape into
the tissue and start both an immune response and a healing response. The release of histamine and another mast cell chemical,
heparin, which slows down blood clotting in the area, causes the
signs of inflammation—swelling, increased blood flow (which
makes the area warm and red) and usually some pain. Inflammation and the immune response thus go hand in hand in wound
healing.

Oxygenation of each and every cell of our body at all times is
essential to life. If our oxygen supply is cut off for even a few minutes, we die. The same is true inside our body, where an injury such
as a fracture or an event such as a heart attack disrupts the blood
supply and so too the delivery of oxygen, causing cells and tissues
to die.

Circulation of blood, which brings nutrients, oxygen, a[...] mune cells to our tissues and which takes away metabolic waste products, carbon dioxide, and the products of inflammation and immune activity, must be maintained. We can say that oxygenation and circulation go hand in hand.

Nutrition, which includes the provision of nutrient molecules, such as amino acids, fatty acids, sugars, and vitamins, must also include a host of minerals that are needed for proper cell function.

It is not just sufficient to have some oxygen, some blood flow, and some nutrients. We must maintain very precise levels for optimal health, and our major efforts towards becoming and staying healthy must focus on these three physical needs—excellent or optimal oxygenation, vigorous circulation, and complete nutrition. When any of these is below par, nothing works well, and that includes our immune system. The main physical reason for immune failure is poor general health.

Specific Immune Activities Necessary to Maintain Good Health

A quick introduction to the principle support systems necessary for optimal function of our immune response is useful.

Precise recognition of everything in the environment around the body and of anything inside the body that needs to be removed is the key to good immunity. "Precise" means the immune system can tell the difference between a bacterium that has the potential to cause disease and one that does not pose a threat. It can tell the difference between initially harmless common allergens, such as molecules from cat dander, dust mite feces, ragweed pollen, peanuts or shellfish, and other very similar molecules which do have the capacity to make us ill. When this recognition is precise, the immune system responds appropriately—it attacks and kills the dangerous bacteria, but leaves the cat dander and the peanut butter alone; we stay free of disease and we do not develop allergies.

As mentioned above, we want the inflammatory response to be appropriate, not excessive. An excessive inflammatory response, which, for example, produces so much swelling that blood supply and oxygenation are restricted, will interfere with healing by causing more cells to die and reducing the efficacy of the immune response, so that there is greater likelihood of infection. Interventions which, on the one hand, gently cleanse the wound, and, on the other, gently cool and soothe it greatly improve the rate of healing and the success of the immune response.

Inflammation is a natural response to tissue injury and occurs where the body is fighting infection. Inflammation is a very powerful survival response which sacrifices the comfort and sometimes part of the function of the body in order to get us up and around. It may be so powerful as to either kill us or cure us. There is a lot that we can do to make inflammatory responses more body-friendly. We are less likely to have overpowering inflammation responses when our tissues are very healthy, because they have good circulation, oxygenation, and nutrition. We are also less likely to experience life-threatening or overwhelming inflammatory responses when our immune systems are working as they should.

GOOD BEGINNINGS—FACTORS WHICH AFFECT
THE EFFECTIVENESS OF THE IMMUNE SYSTEM

The Birth Experience

Mother's body is the source of almost all the immune information a newborn baby needs. Antibodies from mother's milk and organisms in and on her body instruct the newly-arrived baby as to what it will find in its environment and also provide the first installment of natural bowel flora for the digestive tract.

As a baby is being born, it passes down the vaginal canal and takes into its mouth and nose vaginal, and a little later, fecal organisms, which are ingested. A few moments after birth, the baby samples and consumes organisms from the skin of the mother's chest, hands, and breast. This is all very important. Organisms from the mother, even those from her feces, provide information about healthy immunity and the mother's defence mechanisms. They also are characteristic of the environment in which the mother lives and into which the child arrives. Lastly, and of great importance, these organisms become part of the child's digestive gut flora, an essential population of organisms which immediately begin to propagate and program the lymphatic tissue around the small intestine. This intestinal lymphatic tissue comprises approximately 70% of the entire lymphatic and immune tissue of the body.

Inhabitants of the world beyond the mother—the soil organisms and other environmental micro-organisms—will be encountered, consumed, and similarly treated by the child a short time later.

The antibodies passed on to the baby through mother's milk will reflect the immune status of the mother and should represent the immune memory established over the years that she has successfully fought disease in her environment.

It can be very disruptive to the development of a child's immune system if the child does not experience a vaginal birth or is not able to physically contact the mother's skin and nurse. Equally disruptive can be an environment into which the child is born that is foreign to the mother, say a hospital, where most home organisms are absent, but where virulent antibiotic-resistant organisms may be present. A sudden change in environment caused by war, migration, dislocation, and travel also exposes the newborn prematurely to organisms of which the mother has no experience.

Caesarean section, while a life-saving procedure in some cases, is used far more often, for the sake of convenience, than is absolutely necessary. The exposure of the newborn infant to its own mother's vaginal, fecal, skin, and other organisms is an essential introduction for the baby to its mother's body. Also, by virtue of the mother's response to her home and local environment and her successful creation of an effective immune relationship with it, the baby will receive advance information about that environment through antibodies in the mother's milk. When this does not occur, the child is at a distinct disadvantage, and studies have shown that children that did not experience vaginal birth have more immune problems later in life and also, oddly enough, a higher incidence of behavioural problems.

Breast-Feeding

Breast-feeding is important for several reasons. The organisms encountered in breast-feeding contribute to the bowel flora, and the antibodies in that breast milk establish the first elements of the infant's immune response. The nutritional make-up of mother's milk is perfectly suited for the complete nutrition of the baby. Prepared infant formulas, made from cow's milk or soy, have been modified to resemble mother's milk as closely as possible. However, these formulas are so highly processed that, while they may contain all the essential nutrients, they actually possess very little vitality. Furthermore, these infant formulas often contain residues of bovine or soy lectins, effecting not only indigestion (colic) but also overstimulation of the infant's immune system and overload of the immature digestive system, causing inflammation. It should also be mentioned that bovine lectins are antigenic to most blood types.

It is common practice to store expressed breast milk for feeding when the mother is not available. While there is no problem in storing breast milk for later use, it is important not to microwave this milk, since the valuable antibodies are totally destroyed by both microwaves and heat.

The value of breast-feeding as a bonding activity is difficult to evaluate objectively, but there are no doubt many benefits.

Birth environment is important to the establishment of the young immune system. Studies have shown that babies born in hospitals have inferior colon microflora. These babies' gut flora contain fewer of the beneficial organisms needed to stimulate the intestinal lymphoid tissue and more pathogenic organisms, which make the baby more susceptible to disease at that time and later in life.

A Child's Environment

In addition to the factors mentioned above, it is important to introduce children to their environment in a balanced way. A homebirth into a naturally clean home is the best start. By "clean" is meant swept, dusted, and vacuumed, with mouldy or deteriorating food promptly removed. Cleaning cloths and washcloths should be regularly washed to prevent the overgrowth of germs. It is better not to use disinfectants in the form of sprays, cleaning solutions, medicated wipes, and so on. While these do kill organisms, they also put pressure on the populations of organisms to mutate and destroy the natural symbiotic relationship that should exist.

There are exceptions. Serious life-threatening infectious diseases, particularly those caused by certain kinds of Streptococci and Staphylococci, may require extra cleansing. Yet even these diseases, most of which are now thankfully rare on account of better hygiene, usually pose no threat if the mother's health and immunity are robust and the baby's start has been a good one.

Stress of a psycho-spiritual nature can diminish immunity. Babies and children growing up where there is anxiety, fear, guilt, shame, and anger are less vital than those that grow up encountering self-worth, unconditional love, security, and confidence.

Stress caused by lack of sleep, poor nutrition, overwhelming responsibility, and trauma also requires special measures to help the mother and the child build the vitality needed to enable the immune system to develop fully and in a balanced way.

IMMUNE FOR LIFE

How the Immune System Responds to Unavoidable Challenges

Epidemic diseases have occurred with regularity throughout history and still do occur from time to time in different parts of the world. There is growing concern about the possibility of new diseases, especially viral ones, and some of the old ones, such as tuberculosis, causing epidemics now. The best defence against an infectious disease, even one totally unfamiliar to our immune system, is a history of successful recovery from illness. It is so important that we expose ourselves to pathogenic, that is, disease-causing organisms on a regular basis, that we become sick enough to fully activate the immune system and then recover. This must happen over and over again, so that our immune system is able to respond to an infectious threat with a rapid and effective result. The immune system can only build lasting immunity in the form of an effective defence against any microbial threat if it has had a lot of practice. That practice must include encounters with a variety of pathogenic organisms—viruses, bacteria, fungi, protozoa, and others. From this there arises a wideness of experience, a fully developed immunity, and the capacity for rapid cellular and humoral responses. Naturally, overall health and vitality are also essential.

Disturbance and dislocation of normal patterns are the major reasons that epidemics are so lethal. Examples of these are:

- travel, which can quickly transport pathogens to areas previously unfamiliar with them.

- changes in diet and other lifestyle patterns as a result of people moving away from their familiar culture in order to escape war, famine, and even the epidemics themselves.
- failure of sanitation and food and water supplies during natural disasters, and so on.

Survival skills that are most effective will include knowledge of how to establish, rebuild, and sustain our immune systems. In times of challenge, when we have done everything else humanly possible, medicinal herbs that can support the immune system can make the difference between life and death. Indeed, a knowledge of the food and medicinal properties of the indigenous plants of an area can save many lives.

How We Maintain a Healthy Immune System as We Age

Natural aging does not create illness or disease. If we are able to look after ourselves with appropriate nutrition, exercise, and access to a natural environment, and if we have positive attitudes and beliefs, we will always be in the process of healing. Healing means that we look for the causes that underlie symptoms on any level and seek to correct them, always trying to come into harmony with nature and natural or universal law. The extent to which we are able to do this determines the effects the aging process will have on us. Certainly there is a genetic factor. Also, the purpose for which we came to earth and the extent to which we feel we are fulfilling that purpose will have a big impact. The fact is, normal aging need not mean disintegration. Disintegration occurs if we do not take responsibility for our health; a failure partly due to ignorance—be it physical, mental or spiritual—and partly due to circumstance.

The more interested we are in becoming in tune with the needs of our body, with the world around us, and with nature, the more inner help we will receive. What is meant by this is that there is a universal law, a healing power of nature, operating inherently within each one of us and known to us in our hearts. As we seek and find this inner dynamic and come into harmony with it, the information we need for good health will unfold for us. What it takes to access it is to desire it in the depths of our heart. The extent of our yearning will determine our success. Strategies based on this principle will enable us to consciously and knowingly improve our health, strengthen our immunity, and in most cases increase our life span.

CHAPTER THREE
The Compromised Immune System

DNA (*deoxyribonucleic acid*) is the molecular material from which our genes and chromosomes are made. When a man and woman conceive, each contributes half of the DNA of the child—the father provides the sperm and the mother the egg. Naturally, the health and vitality of the parents will greatly affect the health of their DNA and the health of the whole reproductive process itself. The fertilization of the egg by the sperm and the first few crucial cell divisions will determine the health of the embryo. The human body has built-in mechanisms whereby severely damaged embryos die off, but even so many babies born are not as healthy as they should be, even though they might not be physiologically abnormal.

DNA is more complex in its functions than simply the selection, mixing, and inheritance of genetic material. Most of our DNA is not genetic in nature. About 80% of it carries information in another form, and recent research suggests that this DNA can be altered by many environmental factors, including the psycho-spiritual environment in which the baby was conceived and in which it develops during pregnancy.

Thus it is evident that, in order for a child to have a good start, the parents' DNA must be as healthy as possible in every way.

Healthy Parents, Healthy Child

The vitality of the mother's egg and the father's sperm is only part of the story. The reproductive tissues of the father, which secrete the fluids that bathe the sperm and contribute to the greater part of the semen, must be healthy in order to have viable strong-swimming sperm. Likewise, the reproductive organs of the mother—her ovaries from which the eggs depart at ovulation, the fallopian tubes where the fertilization occurs, and the uterus itself, where implantation of the young embryo and its subsequent development takes place—must be in tiptop shape.

We cannot isolate these reproductive organs from the rest of the body. If we are not maintaining clean, vital, healthy tissues in our body as a whole, our reproductive organs will not be healthy either.

We have spoken about factors that determine health—everything from good nutrition and sleep on the one hand, to positive attitudes, beliefs, and relationships on the other. All of these come into play before a baby is even conceived. The very poor conception rates in North America and other parts of the developed world testify to our poor general health. Even if we have a healthy conception, pregnancy, and live birth, all may not necessarily be well. Many of our functions and systems may be compromised and clearly are, judging by the increasingly higher incidence of all classes of childhood disease. The immune system, which is the subject of this book, does not escape the devitalizing and unbalancing influences of rampant ill health.

Joyous anticipation should characterize a man and woman's attitude towards parenthood, from the point of deciding to conceive and afterwards, throughout the pregnancy and birth. There will be good times and bad, but without doubt a generally positive approach will make all the difference.

The Importance of Healthy, Natural Beginnings

The benefits of a natural birth and a healthy birth environment, and of breast-feeding and a healthy mother with a healthy immune system, have already been discussed. These factors appeal to common sense and are very significant for immunity and health.

Why is it that we have lost confidence in the ways of nature? To many, the very word *natural* has come to have a negative connotation. Perhaps this is because of its overuse in ad campaigns which suggest that products that are natural are somehow better; regrettably, many of these products are far from natural, and as a result we become jaded. Another complicating factor is that modern society has moved away from nature and created a very unnatural lifestyle. Imagine the effect of introducing "natural" cow's milk—unpasteurized and unfiltered—into the body of a child who has never seen a farm and who has no antibodies against the microorganisms naturally occurring in milk.

It means, therefore, that, while it is imperative that we once again develop respect for the laws of nature and place greater trust in natural processes, we must be careful that the changes are implemented in a sensible and gradual way.

We can have confidence, however, that with proper preparation the natural approach to reproduction, childbirth, and breastfeeding will assure the best beginnings to life-long health. These foundational activities are so important that, with even a little cooperation from informed and health-conscious parents, a more natural approach to them will yield results far superior to what we have come to accept as normal for our children.

Mother's Immune Status and Baby's Immune System

A strong, balanced immunity in the mother is passed on to the child. Where a mother is healthy and has come into harmony with her environment, the one in which, hopefully, the child will be born, a healthy immune system in the child will be the result.

The immune experience of the mother will be passed on to the child—whether it has been a healthy one or not.

Allergies are much more common in our children than in the past. Statistics show an almost exponential rise. Why is this? Part of the reason is that mothers are experiencing more allergies and sensitivities and are then passing on the antibodies to their children, so that in turn the children are allergic.

The same factors which led to the parents becoming susceptible to allergy will also affect their children, who will very quickly begin to develop allergies of their own. The situation worsens from generation to generation, but with a little knowledge this trend can be reversed.

The subject of allergy and allergic reaction is very complex, yet allergy problems and successful intervention and treatment can be discussed here in simple terms, without going into too much detail.

How then, can the actions and choices of a mother-to-be, prior to conception, break the escalating incidence of childhood allergies and sensitivities?

The first step is the careful selection of foods. Live foods, whole foods, and foods that are organic or free-range should be eaten in combinations that provide a balance of nutrients and should be appropriate to a person's blood type—a matter of great importance in this age of compromised and over-stimulated immune systems. Of all the relatively simple lifestyle interventions I suggest to my clients, the strategy of following a blood type diet has shown the best clinical results. As well, the addition of an immune balancing formula like "Deep Immune," prepared by St. Francis Herb Farm, really helps to remove allergies and sensitivities, so that after a few months a mother-to-be will not pass on these problems to her child.

If Breast-Feeding Is Impossible

Accurate imitation of mother's milk is the key to creating an infant formula that is a good breast milk substitute. Formula companies have done a lot to modify cow's milk in an effort to improve digestibility and create a better balance of nutrients. Nevertheless, I believe they could do even better, particularly in the area of increasing the vitality of the milk. Although a product may be shown by analysis to contain all the correct constituents in the correct proportions, it will have less vitality than a naturally occurring product that has not been processed so extensively. I would like to see breast milk substitutes composed of natural ingredients that can be combined to imitate mother's milk quite accurately, but with less processing.

There are some things that may be helpful to consider when full breast-feeding is not possible:

- if the mother is able to provide even a little of the first milk, called colostrum, the baby will get a better start, because colostrum is rich in maternal antibodies.

- if the problem with breast-feeding is that the baby is not latching on properly, then pumping milk will help, even if only supplying a portion of what is needed.

- if a mother is unable to provide an adequate quantity of milk, even that small supply ought to be maintained as long as possible and then supplemented with formula.

If the formula given an infant is not well tolerated and causes colic or other symptoms, such as rashes or foul-smelling stools, make a transition to another type of formula. Do not be afraid to experiment. Get expert help from organizations knowledgeable about natural breast-feeding and alternative strategies.

Baby's First Solid Foods

Every baby is unique, but there are certain principles that can help ensure healthy development of the immune system as well as build good health. The order of foods to be introduced should reflect the state of maturity of the baby's digestive system. Newborn babies do not have the same digestive strength as older babies.

Many difficulties, such as indigestion and associated inflammation, can be avoided by carefully observing how well the baby digests and assimilates food.

The order in which to introduce solid foods should be as follows: mashed-up fresh fruits and puréed cooked fruits, puréed cooked vegetables, and then grains, eggs, fish, and meat, in that order. In each case, I would select foods based on the blood type.

A good age at which to introduce first solids is about six months. The rate of progression will depend on the child's appetite for the specific foods and evidence of good digestion and absorption. Well-digested food will be completely broken down. There will be no bloating or cramping, and stools will pass regularly and easily and will not smell unpleasant.

In cases where a child has not had the benefit of full breast-feeding, a child-appropriate probiotic—a supplement of naturally occurring bowel-friendly organisms—may be given. This should be done in any case where antibiotics have been given to the baby or in cases of severe diarrhoea.

Observe your baby. Your baby will tell you what to do.

The Importance of the Body's Micro-Organisms

Since the micro-organisms in or on our bodies number about 100 billion, they outnumber the cells of the body by nearly a factor of ten.

The relationship between the cells of our own body and the micro-organisms that inhabit our body must be harmonious for optimal health. We rely on these micro-organisms to keep us healthy. The impact of antibiotics and other drugs which destroy the balance of that relationship has a profound effect on immune function. Micro-organisms mutate very quickly when we use anti-biotics and antiseptics or do other things to threaten their survival. Their natural populations then develop new strains to enable them to survive, but these are often pathogenic. Over just the past fifteen years of my clinical practice, I have observed how several strains of organisms which previously lived in harmony with the body have become pathogenic.

Organisms in the digestive tract help the lymphatic tissue of the small intestine create the right antibodies, preparing it for in-fective challenges. Those micro-organisms living in the vagina are very important for vaginal and cervical health, preventing cancers of the reproductive tract as well as yeast and other infections. Or-ganisms on the skin create competition for pathogenic environ-mental organisms. In addition, all the secretions of the body in the respiratory, digestive, and reproductive tracts, as well as tears and secretions onto the skin, contain an immune globulin, IgA. This protein helps to neutralize potential microbial invaders.

When the populations of organisms anywhere in or on the body have been compromised and are out of balance, inflamma-tion levels will increase. Of particular importance is the effect of an imbalance of the intestinal microflora—technically called a dysbio-sis.

Dysbiosis causes inflammation of the walls of the digestive tract. When inflamed, these walls, made up of epithelial cells, can-not contain the contents of the gut as they ought. Under normal circumstances, only completely digested food molecules, such as single amino acids, simple sugars, and electrolytes, can pass through into the bloodstream. When inflamed, the gut wall be-comes "leaky," allowing groups of molecules into the blood stream.

These groups or chunks of partially digested food are foreign to the blood stream, and antibodies are made which make the person sensitive to that particular food.

The Pros and Cons of Immunization

Immunization is a complex and much debated topic, too complicated for adequate treatment here. But there are some important points that should be made, and, while potentially controversial, there is good evidence to support them.

- Infectious diseases killed millions of people, particularly in the early days of global exploration when novel organisms were introduced by explorers or invaders into populations without immunity to them.

- Around the mid-19th century, at about the same time as the first vaccines were being developed, there was a worldwide decline in the incidence of epidemic infectious diseases. This decline has been attributed primarily, by many reliable sources, to improved sanitation and awareness of modes of transmission of disease. Some of these modes included vector transmission, that is, the spread of disease from creature to creature. Malaria and the mosquito are now linked in this way, as are rats, fleas, and humans in pandemics of The Plague (Black Death).

- Credit is given to vaccination programs for the reduction and eradication of many infectious diseases, but that credit may be misplaced.

- Immunization, a procedure the value of which is still being debated, has many pitfalls.

    a) It removes the opportunity for populations to encounter and defeat specific disease-causing organisms. This denies vaccinated people natural immunity to these diseases and the experience of fighting and overcoming them. As a result, their immune systems are not as well prepared for subsequent challenge.

    b) Although the quality of vaccines is reputed to be improved in recent years, vaccination has contributed to outbreaks of disease through contamination by foreign viruses—a likely cause of AIDS—or by using attenuated (not quite dead) organisms which retain the capacity to cause disease.

    c) It may produce partial immunity, and the vaccinated population, if subsequently infected, may develop an atypical and frequently more serious form of the disease—atypical measles is an example.

    d) It may overstress the immature immune system, thereby damaging it, in some cases for life, the result being an impaired ability to respond to later infections.

e) Vaccines usually contain mercury compounds and also traces of allergenic proteins, such as egg.

f) There are many other pitfalls also, too complex and numerous to be included here.

- Once a disease has been almost, but not completely, eradicated in one area, there is virtually no population to infect the child or expose the child, which means that natural immunity to that disease is not developed in childhood. If an unvaccinated child encounters the illness, it will usually handle it well and develop immunity; but, if that child does not experience the infection and contracts the disease later while travelling as a teen or adult, the symptoms are typically more severe.

We are now in a position as a society where it is very difficult to backtrack on the policy of vaccination, even though we know that it weakens the immunity of the general population, particularly with regard to new epidemics.

Herbal formulas can be of great value to correct all of these immune problems, especially when they are accompanied by good lifestyle habits and public policies that promote balance in nature.

The Cause of Inflammation and Its Danger

Inflammation throughout the whole body, affecting every tissue, is called systemic inflammation. This is distinct from local inflammation, which occurs in one spot or in one tissue or organ. Examples of local inflammation would be:

- a mosquito bite, where the saliva of the mosquito is irritating to the tissues, and histamine is released.

- toxic doses of a chemical, such as carbon tetrachloride, which has been used in dry cleaning, are processed by the liver, causing liver inflammation.

- we twist our ankle—tissues are torn and a strong inflammatory response soon follows. Typically, we slow this down by the application of cold packs.

In reality, whenever there is a local inflammation, some of the mediating chemicals enter the bloodstream and cause mild systemic inflammation. Digestive inflammation, particularly if chronic, can and does cause body-wide inflammation. The contributors to this are:

- poor digestion of foods, which may then putrefy or ferment; the inflammatory products of this process cause local inflammation, such as a swollen belly from swollen intestines, and subsequent systemic inflammation.

- inappropriate foods, meaning:
  a) foods to which a person has antibodies characteristic of his blood type.
  b) food additives, which are not foods at all, and which cause irritation in a sensitive person and eventually an immune response.

c)   foods to which a person is sensitive for reasons not related to blood type.

- dysbiosis, that is, an imbalance of intestinal microflora.

The significance of this systemic inflammation is that it often causes symptoms such as fatigue, foggy-thinking and reduced mental functioning, headaches, and a host of non-specific symptoms, all of which disappear when the condition is corrected.

One of the most enjoyable aspects of a naturopathic clinical practice is listening to people describe how much better they feel. They speak of having more energy, being more alert, happier, more relaxed, more flexible, lighter—the list goes on. The symptoms of fatigue, slow thinking, low mood, tension, stiffness, and a heavy, lethargic feeling are so common nowadays that people rarely come to be treated for them. They come for a more serious reason, such as abdominal pain or inflammatory bowel disease, but, in the process of treating these conditions, they are relieved of the symptoms of chronic systemic inflammation and feel much better.

Of special relevance to the subject of immunity is that inflammation both compromises immune function and increases the likelihood of cancer in any tissue which is otherwise stressed. The immune effects include a reduced ability to respond as well as an increased likelihood of sensitivities and allergies.

The Effect of Prescription Drugs on Immune Function

Dysbiosis and leaky gut syndrome can be produced in a healthy person of any age by a course of antibiotics. Antibiotics were used very frequently until it was realized that micro-organisms could mutate faster than we could develop new antibiotics to kill them. The effect of this upset to the bowel flora has been discussed already, and its ramifications are broad, extending well beyond its well-documented destructive effects on the immune system. Fortunately, a dysbiosis can usually be corrected by the diligent application of probiotic therapy combined with attention to diet and herbal remedies to heal the gut wall. Once again, immune-active herbs are invaluable here to reduce immune imbalances and the inflammations that are a consequence of sensitivities and allergies.

Some drugs—steroidal anti-inflammatories, for example, such as Cortisone-like drugs—are often used specifically to suppress the inflammation caused by immune activity because they are known to have a direct immune-suppressant action. They also suppress healing and cell-division and increase susceptibility to infection. While the drugs in this class are often life-saving, the body quickly becomes dependent on them, which makes weaning off them difficult. A lot of immune damage can result in the meantime.

Other classes of drugs are used deliberately to suppress the immune system in organ transplantation. Cancer treatment drugs have as strong an effect on bone marrow and lymphatic tissue as on any rapidly dividing cells, with a predictable reduction in immune capacity.

Alternative treatments, such as herbal remedies which can treat symptoms without suppression of the disease or depression of normal function, are preferable. This is another example of trusting the body's own self-healing mechanisms. It is important, however, in our modern age of poor health, damaged immune systems, and more serious illnesses, that you seek professional advice before making changes in your approach to health-care.

WHEN THE IMMUNE SYSTEM FALTERS

The principal evidence of a faltering immune system is an increase in the incidence and, usually, the severity of the following:

- infections
- allergies and sensitivities
- auto-immune disease
- cancer

The Infection Gets the Upper Hand

Increased frequency of infectious disease is a sign of a weakened immune system. Children or adults who in their past health histories fought off two or three infections a year now report frequent, more severe infections. It would be abnormal for a person not to show any symptoms of infectious disease. We encounter disease causing organisms all the time and we must respond to them if we are not to be overwhelmed. A good response can vary anywhere from slight symptoms, such as a runny nose, a raspy throat, and a transient fever, to a full-blown disease which, however, rapidly resolves itself without complications. These symptoms indicate that the body has encountered pathogenic organisms and mounted a successful immune response, leaving the person immunologically stronger and better prepared for future challenges.

When the immune system is completely exhausted, any infection is serious and may even be fatal. Sometimes, the immune system fails because of a severe immune-compromising disease such as AIDS (Acquired Immune Deficiency Syndrome). In other cases, a treatment for cancer or organ transplantation may require partial or total destruction of the immune system.

When the immune system is fatigued, we see more frequent infections, indicating a reduced ability to respond effectively. In addition, the person may relapse—that is, they may think they are better, but, if they return to work or experience stress, they immediately get sick again. Other people recover, but only after a longer duration with more severe symptoms. At such times, complications or irreversible damage can occur.

Finally, the disease may become chronic. That is, the organism, often a virus, is not eliminated, and the person cannot return to health. Chronic bacterial infections may be defeated by antibiotic therapy, but not always. Immune support with herbs may make the difference in such cases.

Allergies and Sensitivities

Genetically based allergies are well known. A person may have a full-blown or severe, sometimes called anaphylactic, reaction to a bee sting, a drug or, occasionally, a food on the first encounter. Reactions such as these are relatively rare, but are becoming more common. Subtle changes in the immunity of our parents and of their DNA may account for this. Further, the immune challenge of increasing levels of toxicity in our environment from novel chemicals is a contributing factor. The presence of other stressors— everything from increased levels of exposure to ionizing radiation to collapse of our sense of communal and personal identity—also plays a part.

Leaky gut syndrome, resulting principally from the consumption of foods incompatible with one's immune system and exacerbated by dysbiosis, is at the root of most of the allergies and sensitivities that I see in my practice. These may be rectified by taking the appropriate measures mentioned earlier in this book.

The immune system's misidentification of a benign substance, organism or other antigen as potentially harmful is the basis of an allergy or sensitivity response. This happens principally when our immune systems are fatigued, especially when substances are present in such large amounts over long periods that eventually an immune response is triggered. Fortunately, such acquired sensitivities can usually be encouraged to subside by the appropriate use of dietary, bowel-healing, and immune herbal formula interventions.

Auto-Immune Disease

Auto-immune disease is a more and more prevalent component of our ill-health than ever before. At one time, we recognized a handful of fairly distinct diseases, such as thyroid disease, diabetes mellitus, rheumatoid arthritis, systemic lupus erythematosis, and so on. Now we are finding an endless number of auto-immune components in many diseases and syndromes, such as chronic fatigue syndrome, fibromyalgia, and a variety of so-called idiopathic conditions for which the cause is still not well understood. Various types of arthritis and rheumatism, including muscle, connective tissue (collagen), nerve, and circulation disorders all have auto-immune components.

This inability of our immune system to be precise, to discern the difference between self and non-self, is a serious and deep-rooted problem. Immune fatigue from overstimulation by too many antigens is a clear-cut cause of this. While it is not easy to prove a connection, I feel sure that the increase in auto-immune disease is related to the devitalization of tissues. This may occur as a result of fatigue, the lack of balance in our lives, a loss of connection to the curative elements of nature, and an increased confinement and isolation of the self within the mind, coupled with an ever-diminishing awareness of what is going on deep within us and our separation from natural cycles and rhythms, such as day and night, seasonal fluctuations, and other less obvious cycles. These and other factors which separate us from our true nature—our identity—make autoimmune disease an inevitable consequence.

When we are no longer aware of our body in its wholeness and no longer aware that some part of the self has been in a sense severed or blocked from that wholeness, then we lose connection with those blocked parts of our self. It is then that our own immune system seeks out and destroys such parts, because it seems, indeed, that they no longer even belong to us, but have become non-self. When we are self-aware and connected also to the rest of nature, in harmony with all creation, auto-immune disease is practically impossible.

Immunity and Cancer

Devitalization, a continuation of our theme from the previous section, is at the root of cancer. Devitalization can occur as a result of many factors. Some of these are:

- carcinogenic (cancer causing) chemicals which alter our DNA and change the behaviour of cells, so that they no longer follow the rules of that tissue.

- radiation, which also causes mutations in our DNA.
- inflammation, which, while less intense in its effects on DNA, gradually alters cell metabolism and increases the level of susceptibility to carcinogenic substances and radiation.

The natural tendency of abnormal cells to self-destruct, known as apoptosis, occurs when cells mutate. However, because of devitalization of the tissues—from whatever cause, but especially where there is a reduction in circulation, oxygenation, and nutrition—some important cell functions, such as apoptosis, become compromised. Furthermore, the natural ability of the immune system to detect and repair damage to DNA and to detect and destroy abnormal cells is diminished or lost. This leads to a potentially massive increase in the number of abnormal cells, cancer being only one of many irregularities of function that may occur.

But, how can the body successfully fight cancer? If we knew the answer to this question, we could all rest easier—yet perhaps we already do know, at least in part. To summarize, we will have better results in preventing and fighting cancer when we:

- reduce the factors in our lives which caused the now-cancerous tissues to become devitalized.
- strengthen our immune response to the cancer cells themselves.

Strengthening immunity specifically to fight cancer is of great importance. Cancer cells, while they may still be considered part of self, have changed so much that a strong immune system will respond to them by both cellular and humoral mechanisms. Quite a number of herbal remedies have been shown to be immune modulators and have specific anticancer action. Some of these herbs, medicinal mushrooms for example, such as Reishi (*Ganoderma lucidum*), Shiitake (*Lentinus edodes*), Maitake (*Grifola frondosa*), Chaga (*Inonotus obliquus*) and others, have scientifically proven anticancer activity. Other plants, such as the Chinese tonic herb Astragalus (*Astragalus membranaceus*) and Codonopsis (*Codonopsis pilosula*), have shown specific anticancer activity in well-designed experiments.

The amazing thing is that these same herbs also have an overall tonifying or healthful effect on the whole body while strengthening the balance and efficacy of the immune system.

The Effect of Attitudes and Beliefs on the Immune System

A common and unsolicited response from clients who are taking any one of a number of botanical immune formulas is that they feel better. This is particularly marked amongst those who have cancer. It is not ethical to claim to treat cancer or to offer a herbal remedy with any kind of guarantee. In reality, the cancer treatments of mainstream medicine cannot be offered with any guarantee either, although the results in some types of cancer are quite satisfactory.

What is of interest to me is that herbal remedies, such as the Hoxsey Formula or the Red Clover herbal combination, various mushroom-based formulas, and St. Francis Herb Farm's Deep Immune formula all quite often elicit the spontaneous response: "I feel so much better." There are no double-blind placebo controlled studies verifying this statement. I am sure there are those who would consider such a statement an affront to mainstream medi-cine and, at the very least, an offer of false hope. I cannot and do not make claims that I can cure cancer or that people will be helped. However, I do outline strategies that give people the ra-tionale for a program to increase their vitality and support the im-mune system, eliciting this same positive response.

It is difficult or impossible to measure, however, what actually happens in the person. Many herbalists believe that plants which are supportive of the immune function and which have proven anticancer action also support a return to balance of energy, marked by improved functions of digestion, elimination, and circu-lation. People can feel these changes and remark on how much better they feel. In turn, this growing sense of wellness engenders hope, determination, increased strength and focus, and the will to live. This is a heartening sign—the immune system is working bet-ter!

CHAPTER FOUR
Regaining Balance

SUPPORTING RECOVERY OF THE IMMUNE SYSTEM

To support normal function—this is the *modus operandi* of the holistic physician. Built into every cell, every membrane, every organelle, every tissue, every organ, is the ability to function normally or healthily. This is not something we have to teach the body how to do. Our body, by nature, knows what health is, how to identify disease and how to respond appropriately, so that healing can occur.

A strong vital physical body and a positive psycho-spiritual identity provide us with a landscape of the self and are described as the terrain. The terrain, when strengthened through tissue nutrition, oxygenation, and blood circulation, becomes inhospitable to foreign organisms and will begin to heal. As an essential part of this process, we must also remove or neutralize, in whatever way possible, any unbalancing factors such as weather, environmental toxins, and things that stress us emotionally, mentally or spiritually.

A healthy terrain can be restored and its vitality maintained on all levels by provision of proper support, including herbal remedies. A sick person whose terrain is strong and well-supported will mount a strong immune response, and healing usually follows.

Healing the Physical Body

Nutrition, oxygenation, and circulation will allow unhealthy tissue to recover. Blood, carrying a complete range of nutrients and ample oxygen, nourishes sick cells. This allows the cells to unload any toxic waste products from cell metabolism, which can then be transported to the organs of elimination for removal. This process, called detoxification, transports wastes and other toxic materials away from the tissue to the liver and kidneys, the principal organs of detoxification. The kidney excretes its toxins into the urine, and the liver, through the secretion of bile, sends its toxic load into the intestines. Blood, carrying toxins, also contributes to perspiration, our breath, and even tears and other secretions—all of these help to carry the toxins out of the body.

Sleep allows healing to progress at a faster rate. While we are asleep and resting, our bodies can direct more energy to the effort of cleansing and healing. The healing power of nature in sunshine, pure water, clean air, and earth can also contribute very significantly to healing the body as well as the spirit.

Naturopathic medicine is founded on the principles of Nature Cure, practiced since the earliest days by wise physicians, but carried to the level of a high art and science by European pioneers of healing in the 19th and early 20th centuries. Nature Cure relies on

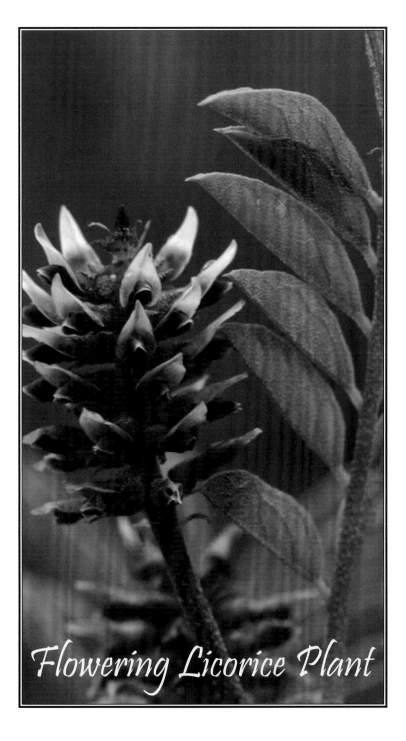
Flowering Licorice Plant

Most of us associate Licorice with candy or sweets. In fact, Licorice is a fascinating and versatile perennial herb that grows mostly in warmer temperate regions. There are at least fourteen species of this plant, whose Latin name actually means sweet root. It is the naturally sweet root that is widely used not only commercially, but for medicinal purposes as well. Licorice has been employed in this way as a medicine for thousands of years in both Western and Eastern cultures. Chinese medicine in particular has held it in high esteem. Traditionally it has been used effectively as a liver protective and immunostimulant, and to treat a range of ailments, including stomach ulcers, abdominal pain, sores and abscesses, sore throat, and insomnia. Licorice is one of the ingredients in an ideal generic immune formula.

the goodness of nature to restore us by providing wholeness and balance, exemplifying the template of good health. Our body carries within it the healing power of nature—a deep knowledge, a blueprint for health. Nature Cure connects us to the healing power of nature as carried also in the very elements of nature around us.

The medicinal herbs, our plant allies, take Nature Cure to another level by their ability to correct our physiological imbalances through pharmacology. Through their energetics, they also restore normal tissue function, reminding us of the universal laws which we may no longer remember or for some reason ignore.

Another essential aspect of Nature Cure is ideal nutrition, the provision of a complete range of nutrients in proportion to the body's needs. Ideally, this nourishment should be provided from a live, whole food source to ensure that all the nutrients are presented to the body in a usable and balanced form. The food should be prepared in such a way that its vitality is maintained, while at the same time the nutrients are made readily accessible. The nutrients in raw food are perfectly balanced in most cases, but often inaccessible because they are contained within cells that the body cannot easily open. Good chewing will help, but cooking to varying degrees is essential to liberate nutrients, especially vital minerals, from many vegetables, legumes and grains.

Live, whole foods are foods that are still whole, as they occur in nature. Foods such as fresh fruits and vegetables are still metabolizing, still alive; a carrot-top placed on a saucer of moist sand will start to grow. Nuts, legumes and grains, freed from their shells, pods or husks, will keep for years while dry, but, if planted in moist soil, will germinate. Animal foods, appropriate and indeed essential for some people, should be derived from healthy animals that have led natural healthy lives—organically raised without the artificial use of drugs or hormones. These foods should be fresh and pre-pared without excessive heat.

Lastly, foods must be compatible with our physiological needs. Traditionally prepared foods and foods that are traditional to our environment are often the best for us; however, transitions to these types of food should be gradual so as not to shock the body. For many, implementation of the blood type dietary guidelines can make a big difference. The importance of a traditional diet to our overall health today is due in large part to the fact that in the course of the development of Western cultures, particularly in this scien-tific age, we have made dramatic changes to the food we grow and eat. Our bodies simply have not adapted quickly enough to keep step with these changes in diet.

Healing accelerates when we sleep. Sleep is another important factor in supporting the recovery of the immune system. There are many reasons for this. During sleep, our level of physical activity is markedly reduced, providing more energy for detoxification, re-pair, and healing. Similarly, while asleep we do not create as many metabolic by-products or waste materials, allowing the organs of detoxification to operate on a deeper level.

Balance is restored during sleep. The destructive effects of sleep deprivation need no elaboration. Sometimes the destruction of health that has occurred in our wakeful state is more than we can correct with normal sleep. It is then that we become ill. Ideally, when we realize we are getting sick, we should take time off to sleep, rest, and recuperate. Research has shown that those of us who do so lose less work-time and perform better than those who stay at work while sick. If we don't listen to our body and take time to rest when needed, we recover from illness much more slowly.

The connection between a good exercise regimen and healthy sleep patterns is well understood. Customized exercise programs which match the type of exercise, its intensity, and duration to the needs of the unique individual will be of the greatest benefit to the health of that person. Exercise, done with self-awareness, helps us to focus on the affected parts of our body. By bringing our conscious awareness and desire to heal to a part of our body, the healing is facilitated.

Patterns of normal muscle contraction and rhythms of circulation of energy and body fluids are disrupted during illness. Appropriate exercise can restore these patterns by removing blocks and re-establishing vitality and thus immunity.

There are many types of exercise, from quiet breathing to vigorous whole-body workouts. With the assistance of your healthcare giver, design the program that really addresses your deepest needs. Immunity will be restored through this. It is good to remember that passive exercise, such as massage and allied arts, can also be very restorative to the immune system.

It is not possible to overstate the importance of matching healing modalities of any kind, whether exercise, herbal remedies, nutrition or counselling, to the needs of the patient. To do this successfully requires very careful listening, observation, and a safe environment, where the person is able to sense and express his deepest feeling about the origin of his problems and how he feels he should best address them.

Vincent Preissnitz had enormous success and attracted tens of thousands of patients to his water cure centres in the Czech

Republic. Water was the principal natural agent used in the 19th century European Nature Cure movement. His therapy was based primarily on the use of cold water applied to different parts of the body as showers, pours, wet sheets, compresses, and the immersion of parts of the body for short periods of time. During the treatments, his patients were fed a simple but healthy diet and engaged in a lot of exercise, walking in the fresh air and sunshine of the mountains. He emphasized loose, free-flowing clothing to promote the circulation of air.

People with ailments of every description enjoyed great healing benefits from this simple, natural approach. Certainly these methods stimulated circulation and oxygenation and provided clean nutrition. Besides which, the healing centre atmosphere was relaxing and far away from the overcrowded, busy, and perhaps polluted, city environment. What Preissnitz and healers like him realized primarily, though, was that within each of these elements of Nature Cure was the template of health—a modeling of the universal laws by attunement to which we are healed.

The Usefulness of Medicinal Herbs

Plants are healers. We think of them as sources of medicine, and, in fact, they have been and still are the origin of many drugs. Indeed, plants heal and sustain not only humans and animals, but each other as well. Plant life arrives at sites where ecosystems are stressed or damaged and starts the repair process. Animals seek out plants not only for food, but also for medicine and use them in a deliberate and systematic way.

Have you ever seen deer reading up on the medicinal herbs in their area? Any elephants visited your local library recently in search of herbal information? Probably not. Animals intuitively know what to eat and when. Put a herd of cattle in a field of weeds, and what do they eat? The ones that support their health. They will sometime eat other plants, but only when starving.

But if animals *know*, why then do *we* have to *learn* about plants and their usefulness? The fact is we don't—or at least we didn't. We may have become a bit rusty, but the people indigenous to natural environments also have an intuitive knowledge of their plants.

Aboriginal societies in balance with their ecosystem rarely recorded their knowledge of plants. Part of the reason for this is that the plants "spoke" to them; that is, the peoples who lived in harmony with the ecosystem of which they were a part knew intuitively how the plants around them were to be used. The healers of native indigenous cultures were given training to help them penetrate into a deeper knowledge and experience of plants. In this way the sacred knowledge of medicinal plants was passed on, as was the mantle of responsibility for healing.

Plants, then, are powerful allies in the quest for wellness and have a strong ability to heal us on all levels. In more developed cultures, this knowledge of plants began to be formalized. In the process, the old reliance on an intuitive knowledge and a harmonious relationship upon one's environment was often eroded. This erosion is more complete in the tradition of Western herbal medicine than it is in traditional Chinese medicine.

Healing the Psycho-Spiritual Aspects of Immune Function

Because the strength of our immunity is in proportion to the degree to which we live in harmony with our true inner nature, and, by extension, in harmony with the greater laws of the universe, we must first develop a deeper awareness of our inner selves.

Harmony is our goal. Harmony with the physiological workings of our body, harmony with the forces and creatures in our environment upon which we depend for nourishment, healing, and models of behaviour, and harmony, ultimately, with the One who is the source of all harmony. I am often uplifted by the many beautiful names that people give to God: Great Spirit, Creator of All, Divine Presence, Father of us all, and so on. Even if we do not acknowledge a Supreme Being and give it a name, most of us would acknowledge that there are laws of nature, and that we ignore these at our peril.

In all aboriginal cultures there is a recognition of the interdependence of all creatures. Creatures includes humans and also things that we call inanimate—rocks, wind, water, plants and air. There was a time in the Western world, a span of one or two centuries, when we believed that the world was inanimate, an object, a resource to be conquered and exploited. Now we realize that the Earth's resources are finite and can be exhausted, and that we are called to a cooperative stewardship of creation, sensitive to the delicate balance of all things. This coincides with evidence both from mystics and from cutting-edge quantum physics—we are connected to everything and we share with everything in some way that force that holds all things in being. Thus immunity can best be described as living in harmony with nature, honouring the Creator of all.

Harmony with all nature and greater harmony with our true inner nature, through self-awareness, help us to change the way we feel about life. Any kind of positive thought, belief or action, lifts our spirits and so too enhances our presence. It has been said, and in truth, that "laughter is the best medicine." To abandon ourselves to a good belly laugh, particularly in the company of friends, releases a lot of tension. It also releases a lot of endorphins, those neurotransmitters in the body that make us feel good. Laughter, smiles of appreciation, spontaneous expressions of happiness—all of these are aspects of joy, the most uplifting of virtues.

How can we increase our joy? By any activity that is positive and that contributes to a higher good for ourselves or mankind. We do not realize how emotions which are self-destructive or destructive to others actively destroy immunity, but they do. When we entertain negative ideas or emotions, they pull us away from the essential harmony of nature and from its Creator. We become isolated from our environment and separate ourselves from the support network into which we were born. Conversely, any positive idea, belief or emotion brings us closer to our natural support network and so strengthens immunity.

We are, however, often embittered, defeated, lost, grieving, alone, planning or wishing for revenge or at least for justice, and consumed by the apparent unfairness of life. Dwelling in such negativity may, to some extent, be satisfying. For sure, it is addictive, and we may fear change, preferring, as we say, "the devil we know to the devil we don't know." Intense negativity may sustain us for a while, but we will, each of us, have to live with the consequences of the choices we make. Unfortunately, these consequences will also affect the rest of creation, and we can all see where things have been going in recent years.

If we could only find it in our hearts to say at the very least, "If I had the strength and I wasn't so afraid of change, of what people might think, of being thought of as weak... If I could only take a positive stand... I want to enjoy health again—physical, mental and spiritual health. I want to be happy..."

If we were able to give voice to even a fraction of this with a degree of sincerity and yearning, we would turn our life around and be facing in the direction of health. Our immunity would start to heal.

Positivity will lead to healing, negativity leads to illness, and a good, positive consciousness will produce positive results. If we extend kindness to people, their spirits are uplifted, their immune system strengthened. If we hold positivity and envision the positive outcome of a project, we will be more likely to achieve our goals and, incidentally, we will also strengthen the immunity of those around us. If we acknowledge and focus positively on a part of our body, it becomes measurably more alive and less susceptible to disease. Conversely, if we withdraw our consciousness, perhaps because of shame, because of pain, because of perceived ugliness, because of fear that something is wrong, we diminish the vitality in that part. Such a part is more susceptible to disease. Its immunity is diminished and before long it will become sick.

We have spent considerable time discussing how the immune system is affected by such intangibles as our beliefs, attitudes, our self-awareness, our use of consciousness and our harmony with the laws of nature. In truth, these are the most powerful influences. Just look at cancer-counselling centres in medical facilities. People practice visualization, come together to support one another and to lift one another's spirits. Why? Because it helps!

THE ROLE OF HERBAL MEDICINES
IN HEALING AND IMMUNITY

Herbal remedies can have a powerful healing effect by restoring the responsiveness, the precision, and the balance of our immune system. All herbs heal, but each has very specific actions which must be matched to the needs of the immune-compromised person. Herbs from different traditions are not fundamentally different in essence, but we may look at each herb differently, depending on our tradition, on account of the unique cultural characteristics which have shaped our view of health, healing, and plant remedies.

We know all plants have chemical constituents, some of which have physiological effects strong enough for us to measure them. Such plants can be classified by their pharmacological effect. In most cases, however, it is difficult or impossible to identify the constituent element of the plant responsible for the action we observe. Nonetheless, traditional usage has allowed us to attribute reliable therapeutic actions to these plants. We may group them, then, according to their therapeutic action, such as immune tonic, immune stimulant, immune modulator, adaptogen, vulnerary, etc.

It is perhaps an indication of the limitations of our understanding that we cannot completely explain how the immune herbs work. What we observe, however, is that the complex interactions of the immune system are restored, and the immune system begins to function normally again.

It has been said that there is a plant for every ailment. It is also widely believed that every plant has a therapeutic use, not as a source of a pharmaceutical drug, but by the qualities it possesses as a whole plant.

Therapeutic action is our attempt to codify and classify the actions attributed to plants. As with any system of classification, it is inexact, just as any attempt to classify humans would always leave out the personality, the uniqueness, and the individuality for which we really know and love a person.

Herbs have affinities to certain tissues of the body. Those we are calling "immune herbs" have an affinity for the immune system, and we will describe their major therapeutic actions. Remember, though, that we have only described an aspect of what the plant in its totality represents and can teach us.

- *Tonics* are plants which improve the vitality in a system. An immune tonic will support both the energy and precision of the immune system. The immune system will work harder and also more effectively. However, tonics are not stimulants; rather, they increase immune system activity from a subnormal level to a normal level.

- *Adaptogens* are herbs that improve the function of the body by strengthening and harmonizing the endocrine system—those organs and tissues that produce hormones. In immunity, we are particularly concerned about adaptogens that affect the adrenal gland, although they also have some protective effect on other glands, such as the thyroid and the insulin-producing cells of the pancreas.

- *Immunomodulators* are plants that help to rebalance the way in which the immune system functions: strengthening weak or unresponsive functions and calming over-aggressive ones like allergic responses, for example.

- *Stimulants* are herbs which boost function, often above normal or resting levels. Such an action can be useful to mount a strong immune response to an infectious challenge; however, stimulants should not be used for too long, as they can cause imbalance and exhaust the tissues they stimulate.

The mechanisms whereby herbs actually work are not well understood—they are complex and many-layered. However, extensive scientific research in many parts of the world has shown that botanical preparations do indeed improve and restore the functioning of the human immune system.

Botanical or herbal preparations have been tested for efficacy by robust, well-designed, scientific experiments. There have been problems, however. For example, a tincture, an extract of the herb made with alcohol and water, can be made in many ways, and the resulting products are not equivalent in either constituents or energetics. The preparation being tested may have been made from a different part of the plant than that usually used. Plant extracts vary according to the parts of the plant used, the time of year it was harvested, the stage of growth of the plant, and the type of soil in which it was grown. It is very difficult, therefore, to compare results, or even interpret results, unless this information is given. Often it has not been taken into account.

Another factor which affects experimental results is the form of the remedy—tincture, capsule of ground herb, aqueous or solvent extract, etc. Frequently, extracts which do not contain constituent elements representative of the healing properties of the herb are used with predictably variable results.

Despite these flaws and the immense complexity of organism-to-organism interactions—particularly in the case of the interaction of something as complex as a plant with something as complex as a person—science has validated the use of many botanical species for immune support.

A COMPARISON OF MAINSTREAM AND NATURAL APPROACHES TO IMMUNITY

In mainstream medicines there are no drugs which specifically support the normal functioning of the immune system, whereas many species of herb can do precisely this. We have described the importance of supporting the terrain of the body through balanced high quality nutrition, good clean water, appropriate exercise, sleep, and so forth. There are many tonic herbs which nourish and strengthen the terrain. An old word, *alterative*, means a herb which assists normal functioning of tissues. Many herbs, while used more specifically for support of a particular organ, have, in addition, an alterative action on that organ. Another old term, *vulnerary*, means a herb that heals tissue. Herbs that have specific immune actions, while also being tonic, alterative or vulnerary, are those which will prove the most useful in building and maintaining immunity.

The concept of suppression—meaning to remove the symptoms of a disease—is very important in any discussion of immunity. Suppression of symptoms means to make the symptoms disappear by using a drug and, often in the process, reducing or eliminating the body's self-healing ability. When a disease and its symptoms are repressed, a natural healing process is left incomplete.

Suppressive treatment may also mean that the causes of the condition may not have been touched. For example, frequently-occurring infections are not so much an indication of frequent exposure to infectious agents as they are evidence of a weakened immune system. In addition, when using suppressive therapy, such as an antibiotic or an anti-inflammatory, we have not supported or maximized the normal functioning of the body's healing ability.

One feature of suppression observed by holistic physicians is that the memory of a suppressed illness remains in the body. There is a cellular memory of the event and, later in life, if the person becomes really healthy and, especially if they undergo a deep cleansing, the suppressed condition will resurface and the natural healing cycle will be completed. This is sometimes referred to as a *healing crisis*.

Normalization, on the other hand, which is the return of immune functions to normal, can be accomplished by a combination of lifestyle changes and herbal remedies to support the terrain. Herbal remedies can be used to induce sweating in response to fever, if this is not happening naturally. Fever is a very important natural response to infection, as elevated body temperature disables or kills the pathogenic micro-organisms. Herbs may have hyaluronidase inhibiting action, which antidotes the bacteria's ability to invade tissues. They can stimulate increases in the numbers and availability of macrophages and blood-borne white blood cells, stimulate antibody production, and increase interferon levels.

In addition to these support mechanisms for the immune system, specific herbs may also be used as decongestants; as anti-inflammatories to improve lymphatic drainage and to reduce swelling; as vulneraries; as demulcents to soothe and to open the airways (bronchodilators); and as expectorants to remove phlegm from the airways. All of these actions improve the oxygenation, circulation, and nutrition of tissue, strengthening the terrain and helping the person feel more comfortable.

Antibiotics, however, may be necessary at times to control and kill bacteria that have established an infection within us that threatens to overwhelm us. The decision to use or not use antibiotics should depend on a number of factors:

- the vitality of the individual and his immune system—rate of recovery is a good indicator of vitality.
- whether a person has the option to rest and do other things to strengthen the terrain and optimize immune responses.
- the person's belief about his body's self-healing ability, his trust in antibiotics, herbal remedies, etc.

Some of the disadvantages of antibiotics include:

- the destruction, to varying degrees, of the microflora of the digestive tract. It is always recommended to reseed the gut flora after antibiotics.
- antibiotics remove some of the experience of recognizing, responding to, and, finally, healing disease. Such circumvention of a full immune response not only deprives the immune system of

experience, it suppresses symptoms like fever,
mobilization of circulation, sweating, and so on,
which are such an important part of the immune
response.

There are a number of efficacious antimicrobial herbal remedies. Thyme and garlic are known to be very broad spectrum and
effective against even antibiotic-resistant organisms. Other commonly used medicinal herbs work effectively against viruses, different bacterial strains, various fungal pathogens, and also parasitic
infestations. Good training, however, is needed for the safe and
effective use of these remedies.

Herbal remedies may also be useful in support of cancer treatment. In choosing a course of treatment, a person should do whatever they feel the most confident will work. This can vary from re-
fusing all treatment to following the entire mainstream program for
cancer treatment and adding additional herbal or lifestyle programs.

One of my clients, after receiving the diagnosis of a serious
cancer, moved to Oregon, built a small shelter in a remote area,
and practiced meditation and other healing strategies. He emerged
a year or two later cancer-free. Other clients of mine have experienced equally good results from mainstream treatment. It is worth
noting that a number of medicinal plants have been shown to be
useful adjuncts to mainstream treatments as well as providing
benefits of their own.

Feeling at peace with a decision about a mode of therapy
strengthens the immune system and also allows the person to care
for themselves without undue distraction, to make other necessary

decisions, and to bring their life into focus, if they so wish. Not everyone with cancer wants to survive. The freedom to be at peace with a course of treatment may permit a dying person the freedom to prepare for and face the end of life in serenity.

While I believe it is important for each person to choose their treatment program, I feel it is equally important, if you are going to combine different approaches, to let the various practitioners know what you are doing. This is a demonstration of respect for them and will help facilitate better cooperation among them, where the practitioners are willing. This cooperative approach yields better results and also disseminates information. We do not yet have a cure for cancer, but even so, many patients defy the odds and get better. We can learn from them and we can also learn from those who choose not to fight the disease, but permit it to run its course. These journeys should be honoured because, when he is supported, a person can heal to a very deep level and come to a place of fulfillment, resolution, and peace, even in the face of his own death.

CHAPTER FIVE
The Role of Herbal or Botanical Preparations in Immune Enhancement

QUALITIES OF AN IDEAL GENERIC IMMUNE FORMULA

A generic immune formula means one with broad application to the population as a whole. Such a formula is, to some extent, a compromise, since it cannot fully take into account individual needs; however, these can be addressed separately with the aid of a naturopathic doctor or herbalist. The ideal generic immune formula should be one that can be taken continuously when needed and that gradually improves the precision, responsiveness, and effectiveness of the immune system—precision, responsiveness, and efficacy being the key words here.

Precision refers to the ability of the immune system to distinguish pathogenic organisms from non-pathogenic ones; to distinguish allergens which are, in and of themselves, harmful to the body from those which are not; to distinguish self tissue from non-self tissue and debris; and to distinguish dead and dying cells and other materials from live cells. It should also recognize and either repair or destroy cells which are becoming aberrant and potentially cancerous.

Responsiveness refers to the ability of the immune system to respond. This is an expression both of general readiness, as found in a healthy, fully operational system, and of experience or preparedness in dealing with the required immune function. A responsive immune system is always ready and working. This is evident in a person who handles health challenges with relative ease.

Efficacy refers to the ability of the immune system to complete the job with minimum disruption to normal life.

We now need to understand the different ways in which herbs act on the immune system.

The Types of Herbal Immune Activity

Christopher Hobbs, a herbalist, divides the immune activities of herbs into three categories: deep immune activation, surface immune activation, and adaptogenic action or hormonal modulation.

Deep Immune Activation: This action can best be described as support for the processes of cell activation, antibody production, and a host of other responses that occur within the immune tissues themselves. These immune tissues include lymph nodes, the spleen, the thymus, the bone marrow, and blood and tissue fluids, which are part of a larger class of tissues known as connective tissues. Examples of herbs which are deep immune activators or immunomodulators are Astragalus (*Astragalus membranaceus*), Tangshen or Codonopsis (*Codonopsis pilosula*), Reishi Mushroom (*Ganoderma lucidum*), Shiitake mushroom (*Lentinus edodes*), Chinese Privet Berry (*Ligustrum lucidum*), and Schisandra (*Schisandra chinensis*). These are all Asian, mostly Chinese.

David Hoffman makes the valid point that, if as much research had been done on Western plants from North America or Europe as has been done in Asia on Asian plants, we would probably have found equivalent herbs in our own backyard. The Chinese have the benefit of a continuous tradition which still commands respect. In the West, however, new paradigms have virtually uprooted the old.

Surface Immune Activation: The herbs that have this action, used more in a Western reductionist way, are antimicrobials and immune system stimulants. Examples include: garlic (*Allium sativum*), Wild Indigo (*Baptisia tinctoria*), Calendula or Pot Marigold (*Calendula officinalis*), Myrrh (*Commiphora molmol*), Echinacea or Coneflower (*Echinacea spp.*), and Usnea or Old Man's Beard *(Usnea spp.)*. While it is true that these herbs are antimicrobial, this is only a part of what they do. Each has extended actions which support the body, the emotions, and the spirit.

In the case of Echinacea, while research findings have been controversial, it has a proven record as an immune stimulant and demonstrates other useful effects, such as inhibiting hyaluronidase activity, thus impeding tissue penetration by pathogens. It also has strong psycho-spiritual aspects, assisting those whose identity has been challenged and who feel on the brink of disintegration. The connection between a sense of identity and immune strengthening should by now come as no surprise.

Adaptogenic Action or Hormonal Modulation: By this is meant that plants affect the immune system in a positive way by supporting various hormonal influences. An excellent example of this action is the tonic effect of some herbs on the adrenal glands. The adrenals are responsible for a wide range of actions, which include balancing electrolytes, reducing inflammation, helping the body to respond positively to stress, and supporting sex hormone production and regulation.

The Efficacy of Chinese Herbs

Immune herbs like Reishi, Astragalus, and Codonopsis also have tonic, nourishing, and adaptogenic properties. By a skillful combination of such herbs, it is possible to create a formula which is balanced for the population at large and also immune specific.

Such a formula should be neither too heating nor cooling, but neutral. Nor should it be overly stimulating or sedating. If possible, it should act to stimulate and support the circulation so as to benefit those who have poor circulation or who have a tendency to be either too hot or too cold. This formula ought not to be too strong for sensitive people, the elderly, or the young, but be supportive to all. In cases where there are issues of sensitivity, a good practitioner will be able to use the same formula by varying the dose.

Herbs have specific affinities for different tissues and systems of the body. The Chinese were especially aware of this. It is the choice of herbs with regard to their specificity which will improve the balance of an immune formula further. It is important to formulate with herbs that have affinities for the specific tissues that are responsible for immunity as well as those that are supportive.

Immune specificity is attained by combining the experience of traditional Chinese medicine with modern research knowledge. It should be pointed out that our concept of an immune system consisting of specific cells, tissues, and organs was unknown to scholars of the Chinese tradition. This does not mean that they did not know how to help a person survive immune challenges. The herbs they used in a rather general way to balance and strengthen have now been shown to possess specific immune functions.

There are, in truth, many ways to put together a formula to meet these criteria of balance and specificity. Besides the Chinese tradition, herbs can be drawn from several other well-known traditions, including Ayurvedic, Tibetan, or Western medicine. In order to blend herbs skillfully, however, it is usually easier to adhere mainly to a single tradition. The knowledge pertaining to Chinese tonic and other immune herbs is fairly accessible, as there is a very long tradition of formulating balanced herbal remedies.

This is not as true in the Western tradition, where there has been greater emphasis on an allopathic or symptom/therapeutic action approach. Herbs in the Western tradition are often combined to "cover the bases" for symptom treatment rather than with any deep understanding of energetic complementarity. This knowledge was undoubtedly present before the Renaissance and the ascendancy of the reductionist or mechanistic way of seeing life and health. Modern herbalists are reviving a more holistic Western herbal wisdom.

Ancient traditions, such as Ayurveda from India or Tibetan medicine, have preserved the finer points of herbal combination and compatibility. This permits a range of choice insofar as which herbs may be used to formulate an immune remedy.

The immune formulation which I prefer in my practice, St. Francis Herb Farm's Deep Immune, is composed of Chinese herbs. I believe they have chosen herbs from this tradition because they exemplify that traditional knowledge of plant synergy, yet also have had a fair amount of Western style research done on their uses and function.

Adapting Chinese Herbs to a Modern Immune Formula

It is beyond the scope of this book to discuss the principles of traditional Chinese medicine, but a few points are worthy of mention.

Deep Immune®, a product formulated by St. Francis Herb Farm®, was created using knowledge from both the Chinese Tradition and contemporary Western scientific research. A good deal of the formula's therapeutic success can be attributed to the fine balance of herbs it includes, a balance which was guided by the principles of Chinese formulation.

In traditional Chinese Medicine, extreme weather conditions were considered to be one of the major challenges to the immune system. We know that we are more likely to get sick when the weather changes suddenly. Spring and fall are two such times, and special remedies were prepared for the change of seasons. Astragalus and Codonopsis were usually included in these remedies.

For the Chinese, as for us, extreme heat or cold, extreme dampness or dryness, and the effects of wind and summer humidity are all considered very stressful. Since these challenges come from outside the body, herbs such as Astragalus, which strengthen the defences of the body at the skin surface, were considered especially valuable. It is not easily explained physiologically how this works, but there is no doubt that Astragalus and herbs with similar actions increase our defensive energy.

My clients who use this formula tell me that not only can they resist the challenges of the weather, but that they are less affected by negative people, noise, and other energetic stressors. These remedies support our spiritual identity and strengthen our "presence."

But what qualities in herbs help to build an effective immune formula? First, proven immune activity. The herbs must be able to support the immune system by making it more precise, more responsive, and more efficacious. In addition to this general response, if we know plants which have proven antibacterial, antiviral, antifungal or anticancer effects as well, then these would be very attractive to us. Astragalus and Reishi both have such specific actions.

The chosen herbs must also support the terrain. Each of the Chinese botanicals featured in a formula like Deep Immune does this very effectively. It is essential to select the ones which both support the immune system in a balanced way and together optimally support the terrain. In fact, some herbs may be included which may not be recognized for any specific immune activity, but which are generally useful in support of the terrain.

Synergy in Complex Herbal Formulas

"Synergy" means mutual support or working together to produce an overall effect which can apparently be greater than the sum of its parts. In a herbal remedy, we are looking for combinations of ingredient which adequately account for all the desired effects and do so in a balanced way. Strangely enough, a good combination will often have benefits beyond those anticipated—a fruit of the synergy of the composite herbs.

In traditional Chinese compounding there was a hierarchy in the formula, in which one herb was usually considered the key herb and was called the "emperor herb." Other herbs would be added to make the effects of the emperor herb more precisely suited to the needs of the remedy. These secondary herbs might potentiate some actions, offset the excessive power of other actions, or add new desired actions not found in the emperor herb alone. These secondary herbs were called "minister herbs." Another layer, "courtier herbs," was often added to aid distribution, digestibility, and taste, or for nutritional value.

Patient response to the formula would allow feedback, and a formula would be refined over time, based on reported results. Although many formulas became accepted in a standard form, many of which are still available even today, Chinese physicians employed an infinite variety of approaches and made modifications to their remedies as they saw fit. This broad variation in approach characterizes traditional Chinese medicine and exemplifies the need to treat each person as an individual. It also embodies the idea of appropriate response to the unique situation at hand.

To summarize, an effective generic immune formula must be precise, responsive, and efficacious. It must heal, support, strengthen, and tonify not only the immune system, but also the terrain. Finally, besides being well-tolerated and safe, it must provide balance, harmony, and stability to the majority of people.

HERBAL COMPONENTS OF DEEP IMMUNE®:
A MODEL FOR GENERIC IMMUNE FORMULAS

Astragalus or Huang Ch'i (*Astragalus membranaceus*)

Astragalus is the "emperor herb" and has the following qualities:

1. Astragalus is an immune enhancer with very
   broad actions.

   - It strengthens a weak immune system, where
     infections are frequent, recurring, and tend to
     become chronic.

   - It is antibacterial and antiviral, activating sur-
     face immunity.

   - It supports both humoral and cellular im-
     mune responses to infection—increasing and
     facilitating macrophage activity, white blood
     cell counts in circulating blood, interferon
     levels, and antibody production.

   - It counteracts immunodeficiency conditions
     such as AIDS and chronic fatigue syndrome.

   - It is antiallergic and reduces all kinds of aller-
     gic reactions.

   - It has antitumor activity, protects tissues from
     damage by chemotherapeutic agents used in
     cancer treatment, and increases the efficacy
     and specificity of chemotherapeutic drugs.

2. Astragalus is an adaptogen, helping to restore fatigued adrenal glands. This increases vitality, energy levels, strength, and endurance, and slows the
   rate of aging.

3. Astragalus supports the terrain.

   - It increases the rate of wound healing and re-
     duces bleeding.

- It supports the major organs of detoxification such as the liver and kidneys.
- It improves digestion and the absorption of nutrients.
- It helps regulate the metabolism, thereby enhancing the nourishment of tissues.
- It warms the body and strengthens the limbs, making a person more tolerant of harsh working conditions and cold weather.

This amazing catalogue of therapeutic actions is partly due to a complex mixture of nutrient and protective constituents. As well, there are molecules and minerals which have specific immune enhancing effects. No man-made drug could even begin to approximate the completeness with which Astragalus supports our immune systems.

Astragalus has been described here in a fair amount of detail in order to illustrate the range of actions that this herb has. Although each of the other seven herbs in Deep Immune is equally remarkable in its own way, I will note only a few salient points of each.

Codonopsis or Tang Shen (*Codonopsis pilosula*)

Codonopsis is a "minister herb." Astragalus and Codonopsis have been used together as energy tonics in many classic restorative formulas of traditional Chinese medicine.

- Codonopsis is an energy tonic particularly supportive of the fluids of the body—blood plasma, mucus, and lubricating fluids on all the mucous and serous surfaces of the body as well as the movement of lymph, urine, sweat and tears.

- It is a sweet-tasting digestive tonic, supporting nourishment of the body.

- It is neutral in terms of temperature. In many ways, Codonopsis is like Ginseng, in that it is an invigorating herb, but more suitable to a generic formula, because Ginseng may be too hot, especially for the young or those already too fiery or overheated.

- It supports and stimulates cellular immunity, increasing both phagocytosis and antibody production.

- It protects the body against radiation and increases the levels of interferon and other factors which counteract cancer.

Reishi Mushroom or Ling Zhi (*Ganoderma lucidum*)

- It is antibacterial and antiviral and stimulates the activity of macrophages and lymphocytes.

- It protects against the effects of environmental or therapeutic radiation, helping to maintain white blood cell levels.

To quote Ron Teeguarden, from his work entitled *Radiant Health: The Ancient Wisdom of the Chinese Tonic Herbs* (page 4):

"Interestingly, a herb now commonly used in Chinese Tonic Herbalism is the most widely used symbol of longevity—the Reishi mushroom. This mushroom is used in all Asian societies as a symbol of health, happiness, wisdom and long life. It is a common symbol in the art of China and Korea.

"The Reishi is, in fact, a true longevity herb. Though historically it has been a rare herb, it has in recent years become much more commonly available, thanks to modern horticultural technology. Hundreds of scientific studies have confirmed that Reishi can be used to build physical resistance to disease and to treat a wide range of ailments.

"Reishi has many benefits, including protection of the cardio-vascular system and prevention and treatment of liver diseases and even certain forms of cancer. No wonder it became a symbol of longevity."

(On a personal note, I would like to share an experience. A little while ago, I spent many hours at a picnic table beside a lake, preparing the notes for this book, and noticed, to my delight, that growing right behind me, on a decaying stump of an old maple tree, were many Reishi mushrooms. I gathered these mushrooms with thanks and am carefully drying them in my office as I write.)

Siberian Ginseng or Ci Wu Jia (*Eleutherococcus senticosus*)

Siberian Ginseng is an exceptional adaptogenic immune herb, supporting, restoring, and regulating the functions of the adrenal glands, the thyroid, and the insulin-producing cells of the pancreas. Extensive research has shown this herb to be a important ally in counteracting the effects of stress of any sort.

As a regulator and restorative of most of the principal metabolic functions of the body, it plays a major role in supporting the terrain.

Privet Berry or Nu Zhen Zi (*Ligustrum lucidum*)

Ligustrum strengthens and restores the vital energy and the nervous system of the body. It is a rejuvenator, naturally helping to keep the body free of toxins and inflammation.

Its immune functions include general deep immune support and the ability to improve the response to infectious challenges. It is antiallergenic and holds some promise in the treatment of tumours.

Schisandra Berry or Wu Wei Zi (*Shisandra chinensis*)

Schisandra has all the qualities of a tonic herb necessary to support and repair the terrain as well as having some powerful immune actions. The fruit has the remarkable attribute of having all five tastes—sweet, sour, salty, bitter and spicy—stimulating and supporting all aspects of the physiology.

- It is adaptogenic, supporting the adrenal cortex and prolonging life.
- It is a deep immune herb, an immunomodulator, which enables it to increase immunity to infectious diseases, prevent and relieve allergies and sensitivities, and improve the body's ability to recognize and destroy abnormal cells.
- It helps to balance immunity, correcting auto-immune conditions.

White Atractylodes Root, Bai Zhu (*Atractylodes macrocephala*)

This herb is particularly useful in improving the nourishment of the body, increasing vitality, offsetting fatigue, and developing stamina. It does this, in part, by supporting good appetite, the digestion of food, and absorption of nutrients.

It does have immune supporting qualities and has been shown to be helpful in resolving certain types of tumours.

Ural Liquorice Root or Can Gao (*Glycyrrhiza uralensis*)

This herb has adaptogenic, immunomodulating (deep immune), and surface immune actions. It supports and restores adrenal and pituitary function, is immunostimulating and antiallergic, and has antiviral, antibacterial, and other antiseptic properties. In addition, Asian liquorice:

- moistens, soothes, nourishes, heals, relaxes, and softens the tissues of the body.
- is a powerful anti-inflammatory.
- has antitumor properties and increases interferon levels.

What Is a Tincture?

A tincture is a liquid herbal remedy made by extracting the herb in a mixture of alcohol and water. Together, alcohol and water are able to dissolve all the medicinal elements in a plant. The alcohol and water, called a menstruum, are mixed in precise proportions depending on the composition of the plant. The ratio of menstruum to herb is also important. Usually the herbs are dried and then ground in order to provide maximum exposure of the herb to the menstruum.

Since most of the ingredients in Deep Immune are tough woody roots or hard mushrooms, they must be ground up in order to allow for complete extraction. Once the medicinal constituents are dissolved in the menstruum, the mixture is filtered to remove the remains of the powdered herbs. This clear liquid is the tincture.

Quality is the main reason why tinctures are preferred to gel capsules or pills. They enable consistency, stability, and the possibility of variable dosing. A good quality compound tincture is achieved when the manufacturer is conscientious about the following:

- good quality herbs—correctly identified, from reliable, monitored sources, fresh, free of contamination, and harvested at the right stage of growth.
- following the correct procedures for tincturing each herb in the formula to ensure the fullest extraction of the constituents.
- precise blending of the simple extracts.
- quality control at every stage of the procedure.

What Are the Benefits of a Tincture?

The presence of a tincture in the mouth—its taste, its unique character, its flavours and aromas—immediately stimulates a healing response in the recipient. This intimate contact with the healing medicine on so many levels can touch a person in subtle but powerful ways. Very often in my practice I will show my client a photograph of the plant in flower and offer a sample of the dried herb to smell and feel.

It is well known that an aqueous extract of a herb, or of any substance for that matter, becomes imprinted with the character of that substance. Homeopathy and flower essences both rely on this relationship. Tinctures, which are liquid extracts, thus carry not only the physical medicinal molecules, but also the healing essence of the plant. This is akin, on the plant level, to our human spiritual identity.

Because it is a liquid extract, a tincture is rapidly absorbed. Holding a tincture in the mouth for a few minutes, as can easily be done if it is diluted in a little water, allows for the absorption of many of the medicinal constituents and the imprint of the constituent herbs' healing characters. This absorption brings the remedy directly into the blood stream, allowing it to bypass the liver. Other forms of delivery, such as gel caps, capsules, and pills, only begin to break down in the stomach and pass through the intestine to the liver, by which time many of the constituents are destroyed or inactivated. Tinctures, once swallowed, are rapidly absorbed, as alcoholic extracts can pass directly from the stomach into the blood stream.

Further, tinctures are administered in drops, which means that the dose can be varied infinitely for patients of different ages, metabolic states, and levels of sensitivity.

The alcohol in a tincture keeps the extract stable for as long as the alcohol remains in the bottle. This means tinctures have a shelf life of many years. Leaving the cap off or loose, however, will shorten the shelf-life of the product, and it may support mould or other undesirable growths as the alcohol evaporates.

In conclusion, the choice of tincture as the form for their herbal formula Deep Immune was deliberate on the part of St. Francis Herb Farm for all the reasons listed above, and this only serves to enhance this well-conceived product.

CHAPTER SIX
Immune Related Conditions in My Clinical Practice as a Naturopathic Doctor

HERBAL FORMULAS IN THE TREATMENT
OF IMMUNE DISORDER AND DYSFUNCTION

I practice family medicine for people of all ages, from a couple that is planning to have children to the aged in the process of death and dying. While there are people who suffer from an unlimited range of health problems who come to my office for health-care, there are certain predominant groups.

I should point out that as a naturopathic doctor in Ontario I do not practice surgery, prescribe drugs, or offer first response medical assistance for trauma other than minor scrapes and bruises. Nor do I deliver babies. My practice does, however, include support in sickness and health during all phases of life.

While the list of conditions from which people may suffer is very broad, and every person is unique in his journey, there are some common categories of underlying causes. The primary causes of ill health are:

- poor or inappropriate diet and lifestyle.
- mental, emotional, and spiritual stress—what I call psychospiritual stress.
- weak or unbalanced immunity.

These categories, it should be noted, are artificial in that the causes of ill health are all interrelated.

Here is a case in point which illustrates this interrelatedness of the causes of ill health. I recently saw a woman who came from the Orient 20 years ago. She has suffered from severe allergies all her life, but they worsened when she arrived in Canada. Her allergies are quite random, but always worsen when she feels anxious or fearful. I could find no pattern indicating a physical cause, so I asked her, "When you were young, did you have a difficult time— was it hard to find anyone to trust?" She began to weep. She had been left to fend totally for herself as a child. Her family was not supportive, and her country was at war.

Having failed to find a reasonable cause for her allergy pattern, I sought a metaphor to explain her condition. Severe allergies are a result of a dysfunctional immune system, which, in turn, indicates a weakened sense of self. I recognized in her story and the accompanying emotional response the metaphor for her condition: a profound feeling of insecurity about or fear of the world around her. She had an adversarial relationship with the world instead of a reciprocal, loving, and nurturing one. This is the metaphor of allergy. I feel her immune imbalance was the result of a lifetime of fear, loneliness, and difficulty trusting, experienced by a very sensitive person.

Another example would be an intelligent and knowledgeable person who deliberately maintains a poor diet and leads a poor lifestyle. One wonders what psycho-spiritual difficulties cause him to neglect himself in this way.

It seems that most cases of ill health are ultimately rooted in the psycho-spiritual suffering of people. As is obvious from my discussion on the nature of immunity thus far, immune problems are closely tied to psycho-spiritual health.

The people who seek my care are generally intelligent, often well-educated, and always thoughtful; they are often seekers of a way that resonates more deeply for them, people who want to understand, to know a deeper truth.

This latter quality is partly, I believe, the result of naturopathic philosophy and principles, and is partly due to the fact that people who seek alternatives to the mainstream must have thought deeply, must be in search of something. These people are already open to examining life at a deeper level and are often open to looking deeply into their emotions, their minds, and their firmly held beliefs about themselves and life.

Immune function has become a central axis around which everything else revolves, because it is about our identity. Our search for our identity begins by looking for answers to the three famous questions:

1. Who am I?—What is my true identity?
2. Where did I come from?—What are my origins, and how do I fit into the larger context of life?

3. Why am I here?—What is my purpose, what am I here to learn, and what am I to become?

Yet even despite the desire and intent to answer these fundamental questions and arrive at a sense of self-identity, we can experience conditions associated with immune dysfunction. However, these immune related conditions, properly understood and addressed, in the spirit of an ongoing search for wellness, will provide invaluable lessons.

Immune Related Conditions

Generally, the conditions related to immunity that I have treated in my practice include the following:

- *Infections.* These are of many kinds—acute, mild, severe, and chronic. Most problem infections indicate a weakened immune system, and this is an area where almost everyone can be helped, often dramatically so.

- *Allergies and sensitivities.* These fall into two main categories for me: those which originated as a result of inappropriate dietary patterns; and all the others. For the treatment of allergies, dietary changes, combined with immune-balancing by way of herbs, are a powerful and effective tool.

- *Auto-immune disease.* These conditions are many and varied and include:
  a) the various forms of arthritis and other conditions with musculo-skeletal and neurological components, e.g., rheumatoid arthritis, sys-

temic lupus erythematosis, multiple sclerosis,
etc.

b) endocrine problems, such as diabetes mellitus, thyroid conditions, and others.

c) a long and varied list of diseases, among
which Sjogren's syndrome, fibromyalgia, and
inflammatory bowel disease occur frequently.

Auto-immune conditions are more difficult to treat than other immune problems,
though the extent and rate of progression can
often be reduced by approaches that include
dietary changes, healing of the bowel, restora-
tion of bowel flora, and balancing the immune
system.

• *Cancer.* While naturopathic doctors do not offer
treatments specifically for cancer, lifestyle and
herbal interventions can often improve the outcome of the disease.

This is a very brief and inadequate description of the immune
imbalances and their remediation, and I have only scratched the
surface. I do believe, however, that many people can make significant progress with these diseases if they are willing to work at it.

Approaches or Modalities of Treatment

There are a number of approaches or modalities of treatment
that I use in my practice. Among these are the following.

Herbal remedies: Herbal remedies (botanicals) are at the heart
of my practice because, in my experience, they can address every

condition, ranging from the most superficial physical lesion to the most profound spiritual pain.

I use Western herbal medicines in several ways:

- by a straightforward approach of symptom/therapeutic action, e.g., Calendula or Pot Marigold petals (*Calendula officinalis*) to heal cut or abraded skin and mucous membranes, or Bearberry (*Arctostaphylos uva ursi*) used as a urinary antiseptic.

- by using the normalizing, nourishing, alterative functions of plants, e.g., Stinging Nettle (*Urtica dioica),* Dandelion (*Taraxacum officinale).*

- by rebalancing and harmonizing unbalanced systems, e.g., Chaste Tree Berry (*Vitex agnus castus*) to normalize sex hormones.

- by employing the energetic properties of plants, somewhat akin to homeopathic remedy, using dilute solutions or very small doses, e.g., Borage (*Borago officinalis*) to lift the spirits, encourage optimism and positivity.

Traditional use of Chinese medicinal herbs also plays an important part in my practice. I use them mostly to balance unbalanced systems primarily through the use of the tonic herbs and immune herbs.

Diet and lifestyle counselling: As I have suggested above, this kind of work usually gives tangible results and is very empowering to the client.

Bodywork: This may include a variety of different types of massage and gentle manipulation. It can be used in conjunction with a knowledge of Chinese acupuncture points and meridians. The act of touching a person is, I find, very healing for them. While it cannot be explained entirely, I believe it is a combination of the experience of being cared-for and helping the person to direct their consciousness to the affected part, relaxing muscles and connective tissues, as well as improving circulation. There is also the intangible but convincingly-researched healing effect of therapeutic touch.

Strengthening Immunity to Infectious Diseases

Persons with infectious diseases that are occurring too frequently or lingering too long can be helped readily. General immune strengthening through improved nutrition, circulation, and oxygenation, combined with specific strengthening and balancing of the immune system by an appropriate immune formula, like St. Francis Herb Farm's Deep Immune, is almost invariably successful.

The result is an increased resistance to infectious disease as shown by reduced frequency, and when infection occurs, such people develop only mild symptoms (e.g., brief fever and malaise). They experience a rapid and complete recovery from infectious diseases which have penetrated the body's defences, where previously a more severe or prolonged illness would have been typical.

There is growing concern nowadays about the increasing prevalence of powerful new strains of viruses and antibiotic-resistant bacteria. Our best defence against such organisms is to build a strong terrain as well as a strong, experienced immune system. Specific herbal remedies can be combined with lifestyle changes to build a healthy terrain.

Herbal remedies like Deep Immune target the immune system directly and build and restore it in all its aspects. Because these herbs also have energetic properties which can support a person at every level, the action of Deep Immune provides the ultimate enhancement of the whole immune system in a person who is willing to cultivate positive attitudes. Herbal remedies like this are also known to have specific antiviral, antibacterial, and antifungal properties among others, which serve to protect us further from these potentially dangerous challenges.

Treating Allergies and Sensitivities

Today, so many people, including children, suffer from allergies and sensitivities. Herbal remedies can be of great help in these cases too. In any discussion of allergy issues, there are key elements that need to be addressed. These are:

- diet, digestion, bowel health, and bowel flora.
- the fear, isolation, mistrust, and other attitudes and emotions which separate people from the healing power of nature.
- the immune system itself.
- protection of the person from toxic and irritating chemicals in our environment. Of critical importance is the provision of organically-grown foods free of pesticides, live whole foods free of preservatives, dyes, and other unhealthy chemicals in addition to the selection of more fibre-rich foods. It is also helpful to remove from our immediate environment irritants such as household chemi-

cals, dust and dust-mites, and animal products
such as wool or feathers, if these present a problem. Clean spring water, fresh air, and sunshine
are essential. These strategies reconnect people to
the healing power of nature around them.

Herbs which are deep immune activators and adaptogens can
address both the second and third points above. Their principal
strength lies in the ability to address the physiological functioning
of the immune system itself, although the energetic effects of these
herbs are also of great importance.

Overcoming Auto-Immune Disease

Auto-immune disease is the fastest-growing class of disease.
Once again, herbs can be immensely helpful. But what is auto-
immune disease? Auto-immunity is self-destruction. It means, in
fact, that our own immune system has mistakenly begun to attack
our self tissue. We may blame these problems on genetics, and indeed some auto-immune diseases seem to be partly inherited, or at
least the tendency to them is inherited. At the risk of being pro-
vocative, I feel I must pose some difficult questions:

- Why or how has the immune system become de-
  ranged?
- Why has the immune system targeted the particular system, organ or tissue that is affected by the
  disease?
- Are there any parallels to be drawn between the
  nature of the disability that our illness is causing

and our patterns in behaviour, emotions or beliefs?

To answer the first question is not easy, but the imbalancing
effects described in Chapter 3 certainly contribute to, and may entirely explain, the origins of auto-immune disease. One way or another we have lost our way, lost ourselves, and damaged our relationship with creation and our fellow creatures.

The second question suggests that the part of the body
stricken by disease is no accident. Since it is the natural state of the
body to be healthy, it follows that the body would only start to destroy itself if the part affected had become somehow alienated and
was no longer properly sustained. The healing arts of massage,
therapeutic touch, visualization, and prayer all testify to this. Each
of these approaches helps reintegrate the body part, so that it sends
the right signals to the immune system. Deep Immune, or a similar
formula, supports a return to normal of the immune mechanisms
themselves, and healing begins.

To answer our third question we must search deeply. All ancient forms of medicine make connections between the part damaged and the state of the person's psyche. In more recent times,
many books have been written for the lay person that set out some
of these correlations. On many occasions I have watched as one of
my clients has made this connection for themselves and is pro-
foundly changed. Balance is on its way to being restored, and often
healing is almost instantaneous.

Supporting Cancer Treatment

In all cases, naturopathic doctors try to understand and treat
the causes of disease. However, as the incidence of cancer contin-

ues to rise, it poses a unique dilemma, for, while the direct physiological causes of this disease are not always well understood, many of the risk factors are. We must address these risks, often encouraging people to change habits and lifestyle choices to the extent they are willing to listen, as well as supporting better general health and better immunity in those with cancer.

Removing known causes of cancer is essential. The links between smoking and cancer, radiation and cancer, asbestos and cancer and a host of other chemicals and cancer are all well documented. We also know that the mutations which lead to cancer are constantly healed in a healthy body with a healthy immune system.

It is vital to keep the body clean, free of toxins, whether from outside the body or from within, generated by poor digestion, poor bowel health, stress or negativity. Vital also is the use of immune herbs, which help optimize immunity, while at the same time providing the benefit of their built-in cancer-fighting properties.

WHAT A NATUROPATHIC DOCTOR LOOKS FOR IN A HERBAL IMMUNE FORMULA

To summarize what has already been explained earlier in this book, an effective, safe, and generally applicable or generic immune formula must:

- be made from top quality ingredients.
- be compounded from herbs known to have the specific immune actions required.
- be balanced in its actions, as a result of skilled compounding by the manufacturer.

- be extracted correctly to ensure that the healing actions of the herbal ingredients are optimally available.
- be consistent from batch to batch.
- contain no elements that would be contraindicated at different ages or in varying states of health. Care should be taken to ensure that the ingredients will not react with the majority of prescription drugs. Trained naturopathic doctors and herbalists will have studied such interactions, which are, in fact, comparatively rare for this type of product.
- be produced under conditions that fulfill the requirements for quality control.
- demonstrate a consistent and long-term track record of safe, successful use.

This final point is of high importance to me personally. I have no reservations in stating that the St. Francis Herb Farm product, Deep Immune—mentioned frequently throughout this discussion of immunity and formerly known as Astragalus Combination—fulfills all of these criteria. I have given this product to my clients on thousands of occasions and continue to do so because it is a very valuable remedy. It is a great contribution to the process of healing our varied immune problems. While I use a number of immune herbal formulas, Deep Immune is the one I use most often.

Allow me to illustrate how I use Deep Immune by describing a few generic cases:

A thirty year old man with a demanding office job has suffered five upper-respiratory infections in the past three months. This is new for him. He has not yet fully recovered from his last infection, which was probably a viral influenza, and he still has a cough and feels fatigued. History-taking and examination reveal that he has been working long hours, has not been sleeping well, and as a result of the pressure has not been able to cook wholesome meals.

Listening to his chest, I hear some raspiness and amplified sounds in the trachea and primary bronchi, and he describes tightness and discomfort when he takes a deep breath or after coughing.

According to the practice of Traditional Chinese Medicine, pulse and tongue diagnosis reveal that his kidney energy, particularly his kidney yin energy and kidney essence, are depleted and his lung pulse is wiry and depleted.

My approach:

- Strengthen the kidney essence and kidney energy, especially kidney yin, with Chinese tonic herbs. This will increase his energy and vitality. There are formulas which combine tonification of kidney yin energy with tonification of the lung.

- Provide Western herbs which soothe, heal, and open the airways and which act as expectorants, helping to remove phlegm.

- Offer advice on rest, recreation, exercise, and diet, and encourage him by saying that his energy will soon start to improve. This makes following my advice easier.

- Restore immune function with Deep Immune.

In a few weeks, the man was feeling much better and had not been sick again. I recommended that he continue Deep Immune for a total of three months. Later checkups showed a very satisfying result.

In another case, a fourteen year old woman, a competitive athlete, has been increasingly fatigued over the past year. During the last few months she has experienced abdominal pain after eating, no matter what she eats. The pain is in her mid-abdomen. History-taking reveals that as a child the teenager had eczema behind her knees and in the creases of her elbows, and at that time it was realized that the symptoms were relieved by reducing her intake of wheat and dairy products from cows. Abdominal examination reveals tenderness over the small intestines. She explains that it is not unusual to get abdominal cramps and have loose stools. She also feels swelling of her abdomen, "as if I were six months pregnant."

I conclude that her abdominal tenderness and swelling is due to chronic intestinal inflammation caused by general food sensitivity. This generalized food sensitivity is caused by leaky gut syndrome from the inflammation. Her fatigue is a result of her over-taxed and reactive immune system.

My approach:

- Ask her to eliminate wheat and dairy foods from cows from her diet and to follow the diet for her blood type—in her case Type "O"—while still avoiding any particularly troublesome foods.
- Support bowel healing with a mixture of vulnerary, antiinflammatory, and spasmolytic herbs.

- Re-seed the bowel with a suitable probiotic of human microflora.
- Strengthen kidney essence and energy with tonic herbs according to the practice of Traditional Chinese Medicine.
- Treat the oversensitized, exhausted, and allergic immune system with Deep Immune in order to rebalance it.

This program was instituted a step at a time, starting with the first, second, and fourth items. Within a month, her energy was returning. She had a flat and comfortable abdomen. After three months I suggested she try to reintroduce foods that were appropriate to her blood type, but which had caused a problem before. She tolerated them well, an indication that the immune system was becoming rebalanced and the bowel healed. This young woman went on to recover her full health, but remained sensitive to wheat and dairy—a situation that I have come to regard as normal for most Type "O" individuals in our modern environment.

In yet another case, a twenty-four year old woman reports she has been experiencing muscle and joint pain for several months. She has experienced fairly severe pain in a number of joints, particularly of the arms and hands, on several occasions. She has recently been diagnosed with Systemic Lupus Erythematosis (SLE) and has antinuclear antibodies characteristic of that condition. The woman is very hard-working, but vocal about her unhappiness with her life.

My approach:

- Provide nervine tonic herbs to help calm her, lift her spirits and create some hope for the future.

- Plant the seed in her mind that, if and when she is ready, we should look at why she feels so negative and see how we can help her change this.

- Balance her system according to Traditional Chinese Medicine with appropriate Chinese remedies.

- Use Deep Immune to help rebalance the immune system, which had begun to attack her tissues through auto-immunity.

Fortunately, this woman came to me in the early stages of her illness and was proactive and willing to explore any avenue that might help. Her progress was remarkable. Within a few weeks, she was symptom-free, and subsequent blood tests revealed that her antinuclear antibodies had subsided. She did experience one mild flare-up after we started to work together, but this was controlled with a prescription anti-inflammatory.

Later, we pursued the psycho-spiritual aspect, and she gradually realized that she could indeed be a positive person and took steps to support herself with self-affirming activities.

These cases are composite cases, simplified for clarity and brevity, but the process and results are typical of many such clients.

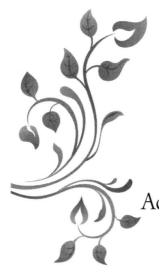

CHAPTER SEVEN
The Seasons of the Year and the Seasons of Life: Advice from a Practitioner

FREQUENTLY ASKED QUESTIONS
ABOUT HERBAL REMEDIES

There are many warnings cautioning people about using herbal remedies. How safe are they?

Foods, especially fresh organic fruits and vegetables, are very safe. It would be difficult to overdose on them. The same is true for most herbal remedies. Many medicinal herbs, such as peppermint, ginger, garlic, sage, and others, are sold as foods, and in these instances we've never been concerned about toxic overdose. Most traditionally used medicinal herbs, while not consumed as foods—usually for reasons of palatability—are equally safe. There really is no distinct line separating food plants from medicinal plants.

There are herbs, however, which contain significant amounts of certain chemical compounds that are pharmacologically active in the body. This means that they will affect the functioning of a physiological process. It is important to be knowledgeable about the correct dose level when using these herbs. Standard herbal textbooks, available at most local libraries, will explain these things and suggest doses as well as any cautions or contraindications.

Certain herbs do have some substances in levels high enough to negatively affect our physiology. We call them poisons. While they can be useful where pharmaceutical drugs are not available, expert knowledge is needed in order to use them safely. Most such poisonous plants have a place in the homeopathic *materia medica*, where the preparations are almost purely energetic and contain little or none of the toxic material.

Humans have co-evolved with other creatures on our planet Earth. Our co-evolution with plants has led to a relationship that has great healing capacity. I feel I should reiterate that there is, in fact, a plant for every ailment from which mankind suffers, and no plant is without medicinal value.

What about when I'm pregnant? Or about to give birth? Can I take Deep Immune or other immune herbs at those times?

Pregnancy is powerful. When a woman becomes pregnant, it seems that her body and even her temperament begin to change in ways that are new for her. Strong, sometimes unfamiliar or unpleasant, sensations flood her body. Morning sickness is a common experience. Most women, however, feel the power of the new experience in very positive ways, developing a greater depth of communication with themselves on all levels of being and often with the new life growing within them.

Respect for this process leads most herbalists and naturopathic doctors to step back and observe, acting only when there is an indication of a definite need for support. Some herbs, such as Red Raspberry (*Rubus idaeus*), are known to support a healthy pregnancy and may be taken by a woman while she carries her unborn child. Certainly, if help is needed, there are herbs of great value in cases of threatened miscarriage or to aid the birth or breastfeeding.

There is nothing in Deep Immune that would be dangerous to mother or child during pregnancy, and so it could be used if needed. However, I do not recall ever having to recommend immune herbs for a woman during pregnancy. In my experience, most women become much healthier during this time, and often their previously bothersome ailments disappear.

What about the use of Deep Immune while I'm breast-feeding?

Deep Immune and most other immune and tonic herbs can be used safely by a breast-feeding mother. These herbs may be useful to support you if you are tired or run-down, or if you and your baby are exposed to infections.

Fatigue is something almost every new mother experiences. Deep Immune and other immune-supporting and tonic herbs can be very helpful for a mother, especially if she is experiencing a lot of stress.

Since a breast-feeding baby usually receives no other food, we generally treat the baby by treating its mother. This works very well because, as the mother's health improves, she is better able to look after her child. Not only this, but, by nursing, the mother passes on to her baby the antibodies of a healthy or healing immune system, and, in the milk, some fraction of the herbal remedy is given to her child.

Exposure to infection is something many parents fear; but, more often than not, this won't have an adverse effect on the healthy baby, since it is well protected by its mother's antibodies passed on in the breast milk. In the case of exposure to more virulent micro-organisms—that is, very pathogenic or disease-causing ones—it may help to administer herbs to the baby as well as the mother. This kind of exposure might occur during hospital visits, for example, or when sick friends or relatives visit, or if the mother becomes very sick herself. While the mother can strengthen her resistance by the use of surface acting immune herbs (see Chapter 5), both the mother and the baby can take deep immune active herbs. A few drops of Astragalus extract appropriate to the baby's weight will help.

Would you recommend Deep Immune for children or the elderly?

While a baby is breast-feeding, it is rarely necessary to treat it, provided the mother is well. Later, as the baby begins to receive solid foods and is weaned, other factors, such as the baby's diet, emotional surroundings and so forth, contribute to the further development of the child's immune system in positive or negative ways.

Children who are often sick may need their immune system supported from an early age and can derive much benefit from a simple herbal regimen. Deep Immune for Children, a formula created by St. Francis Herb Farm specifically for children, is extremely effective in this regard. This mild formula contains herbs that are known to be suitable and effective for children and includes child dosing information on the label. On the other hand, if the growing child experiences an inordinate level of stress in his or her life, then St. Francis Herb Farm's original Deep Immune formula should definitely be considered, since it includes herbs that specifically support the functioning of the adrenals. It is a general tonic formula which enhances the vitality of other organs and systems as well and is safe enough to be used by the young to good effect.

CHILDREN'S DOSAGE GUIDELINE FOR DEEP IMMUNE ®

Age in Years	Daily Dose*
9-14	0.5-1.3 ml (15-40 drops) 3-4X daily
4-9	0.3-1 ml (10-30 drops) 3-4X daily
2-4	0.3-0.5 ml (8-15 drops) 3-4X daily
Under 2 years	As directed by health care practitioner.

*Dose should be taken in a little water on an empty stomach.

The elderly can benefit greatly from Deep Immune. I am constantly delighted at the rapid and dramatic improvement in general health that older people often demonstrate when supported by herbal and other naturopathic care. The effect of tonic herbs specifically chosen for each individual is gratifying, and Deep Immune is exceptionally useful in setting those who have been struggling with immune-related illnesses on the path to healing. Vitality is the key to successful old age. I feel our elders are often neglected, and, in such cases, a little help goes a long way.

DEEP IMMUNE ® DOSAGE GUIDELINE FOR THE ELDERLY

Age in Years	Daily Dose*
60 and over	*0.8 ml (25 drops) three to four times daily*

Should I be concerned about interactions between Deep Immune and any other herbal remedies or food supplements I am taking?

Negative interaction between the herbs in Deep Immune and other herbs is very unlikely. Deep Immune is a remedy consisting of eight herbs, each of which is present in small amounts. In combination they have a nourishing and balancing effect. The most likely interaction would result from someone taking additional tonic herbs, perhaps inappropriate for their makeup, which might tend to work against the balancing effect of Deep Immune.

The total dose of a herb is important. If a person is taking one or more herbal supplements, there may be too much of one or more herbs, creating an imbalance. The results are not serious, but a person may become, for example, too stimulated and unable to sleep. Reactions between tonic or immune herbs and balanced vitamin and mineral supplements, however, are unknown to me.

My biggest concern is possible danger from taking herbs with prescription drugs. What do you advise?

Prescription drugs are given primarily to correct symptoms of a diagnosed illness or malfunction of the body. Many people suffer from illnesses where there is no alternative to drugs. Insulin-dependent diabetes mellitus, post organ-transplant surgery, and surgical removal of the thyroid gland would be some long-term examples. There are other acute conditions for which drug intervention is necessary to save lives and reduce suffering. Many possible complications for which medical intervention is necessary may also occur in pregnancies.

We have the necessary knowledge to prevent most of our medical conditions from occurring, and this is indeed one place where "an ounce of prevention is worth a pound of cure." Unfortunately, the relevant knowledge is not well disseminated, and the will to take responsibility for our health is often weak or absent. Thus serious or life-threatening problems, which require drug treatment, do occur.

If you are taking drugs of any kind, over-the-counter or prescription, you should always tell your herbal or naturopathic practitioner about them. Properly qualified N.D.'s will know about possible interaction with botanical remedies and can advise you.

Cooperation between mainstream doctors and naturopathic doctors, herbalists, and other complementary health professionals is often limited by misunderstanding. While M.D.s are generally not trained in the methods of naturopathic medicine, naturopathic practitioners are given extensive training in mainstream medicine, and so the onus is on them, at present, to negotiate the challenging area where natural medicine interfaces with our present forms of mainstream reductionist medicine.

It would be of great benefit to all if M.D.s and the so-called complementary and alternative medical professions could cooperate for the highest good. In the meantime, keep your N.D. or herbal physician informed of what you are doing and do not mix pharmaceutical drugs and powerful herbal remedies, unless you have enough accurate information to do so safely.

Is there a role for immune herbs in the treatment of cancer?

While medical doctors have generally been concerned that herbal remedies might interfere in a negative way with mainstream cancer treatments, such as chemotherapy and radiation, recent studies have shown that Astragalus, Reishi, and other immune herbs have a positive effect. These botanicals both enhance the efficacy of mainstream treatments and reduce their side-effects.

It would be totally irresponsible to suggest any protocol for cancer treatment here. Strictly speaking, cancer treatments involves surgery, chemotherapy, and radiation—all of these lie outside the scope of naturopathic medicine and complementary and alternative medicine. It is very important, however, in the best interest of those suffering from cancer, that more research be done to see how M.D.s and practitioners of complementary and alternative medicine can combine their knowledge and skills to improve the outcome of cancer treatment, improve survival rates, and also reduce the unpleasant side effects of mainstream treatments.

Herbal remedies have proven anticancer effects, but the research on the integration of herbal and mainstream approaches to cancer is still in the earliest stages. The emphasis at present should be on prevention, strengthening the terrain, and balancing and restoring immune function, which has been the purpose of this book.

What advice do you give to your clients who are also under the care of medical doctors?

Sensitivity to the faith that people have in mainstream medicine and their commitment to it is my first priority. This is true for any health-care discipline, no matter what my personal opinion may be about any particular therapeutic approach. My task is to facilitate healing. While I may point out any dangers I perceive in what a client has chosen to do, I will always try to be respectful.

Negotiation with a client in an atmosphere of respect must be combined with their honestly informing me of their other health related activities. I can only counsel clients according to my level of knowledge about their condition and current modes of treatment. I must point out to them that there are always difficulties when combining more than one health discipline, especially when one is under the care of two or more health-care practitioners from different disciplines.

Once again, I repeat that I support my clients in doing whatever positive thing I feel will move them towards health. Where I can lend knowledge, experience or appropriate help, I will do so.

What are your recommendations for taking herbal tinctures?

The recommended dose of a remedy is usually written on the container. If there is a range, then you should begin with the low end of the dose range in order to test your response. If you tolerate the low dose well, you can then increase the dose. The reasons for dose differences are mostly related to sensitivity and metabolism.

Sensitive people often need far less of a remedy to obtain the results they need. They may be sensitive in the sense that it takes very little of a physiologically active substance to affect them, or sometimes just the fact that they are introducing something unfamiliar into their body requires a period of adjustment. Some people are intolerant of any new substance.

In the case of a tincture for an average adult, I use doses which vary from a drop or less of tincture per day to a teaspoonful 3 times daily, based on a client's sensitivity and response.

Metabolic capacity is important. Children, while smaller than adults, have rapid metabolisms, so they can generally take more of a remedy per kilogram of body weight than an adult. In the elderly, metabolism is slower, and lower doses per unit of weight are usually indicated. Whether for a child, an adult or an older person, I always try to estimate both the level of sensitivity and the metabolic capacity of the individual before setting a dose. Oddly enough, these factors seem more important than the actual weight of the person in arriving at a suitable dose.

Convenience is important if you want a client to take a remedy properly. Most herbal remedies are taken 3 times daily, and, while the optimum might be one dose every eight hours, in practice it is more convenient to take the remedy before meals. Most tinctures are rapidly absorbed by an empty, hungry stomach, as the acidity aids in absorption.

Most herbal tinctures can be combined and taken together in the same water. If there are tinctures and pills, I recommend using the tincture in the water to wash down the pills. Remedies which are stimulating are best not taken at bedtime; however, in the case of calming remedies, I often recommend a fourth dose at bedtime to aid restful sleep.

Do you have any tips to make it easier for me to take tinctures?

Over the years I have learned some good strategies.

- For school age children, give them a dose before breakfast, a dose with a snack when they come home from school, and a dose at bedtime.

- For working adults, the same strategy is effective, or you can put the midday dose in a bottle with water and drink it before lunch. You can, of course, take your tinctures to work, but be prepared for lots of questions. Many herbal remedies can be put into herbal teas. Put the whole day's supply in a bottle of tea and drink it through the day.

- For forgetful people, it helps to place your remedies on the kitchen counter where you prepare your meals. Or, if you don't eat at home, put them wherever you drink water—the bathroom, office kitchen, etc. If you carry a water bottle, put the remedies in the water. Write "Take herbs" in your daytimer, palm pilot or whatever.

You said "before meals." I eat out—what can I do?

Very few herbs are affected by when or how you take them. If you forgot to take your dose before eating, take it after or during your meal. Just make sure you do take the remedies.

Can I take the whole day's worth at once?

You probably can and without risk of overdose, but you lessen the beneficial effects of having fairly constant levels of remedy in your body.

That remedy tastes disgusting! Do I have to take it?

I hope you can tough it out, because it will help you. Usually when something helps, you will take it. You may not come to love it, but you love what it does. I have found that tastes are very individual. What tastes fine to one is almost unbearable to another. Fruit juice, especially grape juice, can help to disguise the taste. This works well for children, although I find children, on the whole, complain less than adults.

STRESSFUL SEASONS FOR THE IMMUNE SYSTEM

Allergy Season

Seasonal allergies and sensitivities usually arrive at predictable times of the year. Start to take Deep Immune about two months before the onset of symptoms. Most environmental seasonal allergies are spring allergies related to tree pollen or to mouldy leaves exposed when the snow melts, or else fall allergies related to ragweed and later to mouldy leaves that have just fallen off the trees.

True hay fever—allergy to grass pollen and cut grass—occurs primarily during the summer.

Exposure to allergens can occur at any time. You will encounter them wherever they are. For some, their sensitivity to perfume is most marked on their way to work on public transit. Others, sensitive to cat or dog dander, will experience a reaction when they enter the buildings where these animals live. In the case of a general sensitivity to allergens, the treatment approach described above will usually reduce or eliminate the allergies completely.

I am very gratified by how quickly and completely most people recover from allergies and sensitivities. In the course of a treatment program for seasonal allergy sufferers with severe symptoms, the second year is usually appreciably better than the first, and subsequent years are still better. Sometimes, and I cannot explain why, the results are almost instantaneous. Two women, with different immune conditions, who did not know or speak to one another, both recently told me, "Deep Immune really helps me. The minute I take it, my symptoms are gone, and if I forget it, my symptoms return."

One suffered from asthma, the other from muscle pain and headache. They are both only a month or two into programs which I hope will lead to complete recovery, at which time they will most probably not need the remedies any more.

Change of Season

Change of season is the concept, present in many cultures, that the transition times of spring and fall are more stressful than winter or summer. It is the sudden changes that stress us and so lower our immunity. In spring and fall, temperatures can fluctuate widely from hour to hour, or even from one side of the street to the other—in shade a cool breeze can be really chilly, but in full sun, sheltered from the wind, it can be hot enough to sunbathe or perspire.

The best support for your own defensive energy is to wear layers and change them as often as needed to stay comfortably warm. Sweating at such times can lead to chills.

I regularly recommend Deep Immune a month in advance of the change of season.

Candy Canes, Easter Eggs and the Halloween Haul

Candy, or concentrated sugar in any form, reduces the protective effect of the immune system significantly and for a number of hours or days afterwards. One of the principal problems with sugar consumption is its osmotic effect on the mouth and throat. Sugar in chocolate or candy attracts water very strongly and damages or destroys the cells in the mouth and pharynx that normally protect us. You can reduce the severity of this by eating small amounts of candy at intervals and by following the sweets with water, a non-sweetened beverage, or with food.

It helps to reduce the oscillations in blood sugar levels if sweets are eaten near food—before or after, to slow down the absorption of sugar and the subsequent insulin release which reduces our immunity. Further, a good diet of wholesome, live, whole foods in balance will make the occasional sugar binge much less of a threat, as the immune system will be stronger and the terrain much more able to tolerate the challenge.

Immune boosting or immune support by Echinacea and Deep Immune respectively can also help. Deep Immune should be taken a few days before Halloween, Easter, or a birthday celebration, whereas Echinacea can be taken right after. It is quite effective to give a child water and Echinacea on their return from a party and, if they are hungry, some steamed vegetables and grains to balance out the cake and other sweets.

Seasons of Added Stress

We usually get sick when the level of stress changes abruptly, especially if we are not mentally and emotionally prepared. We can handle a steady, stressful workload such as a home renovation, a work project, or caring for a sick family member, if we take on the challenge in a resourceful way. The sudden change when the project ends is often accompanied by illness because we have not prepared for the change. Vacations, especially if they involve travel and last minute preparations, can be very stressful. Significant life changes such as promotions, marriages and births, deaths, loss of a job and divorce, are all very stressful.

Strengthening our immunity is the best recourse. We can do this by pondering on our situation in a very deliberate way and seeking the resources we need both from within ourselves and from outside in order to complete the task, while staying strong. Immune herbs, tonic herbs, and herbs that specifically strengthen us where we feel weak or inadequate will make all the difference.

Often my clients ask me how to prepare for times of stress or how to respond to a stressful time that may have unexpectedly occurred. I have a number of approaches:

- acknowledge the nature of the challenge.
- acknowledge how you feel about it and are affected by it.
- choose—if you have a choice—whether, how, when, and where you will accept the challenge.
- consider the resources you need to accept the challenge.
- access the help and resources you need, both from within, through prayer and meditation, and from without, by way of people, rest, food, money, recreation, and so on.

Specific flower essence remedies, homeopathic remedies, or drop dose herbs will help to address emotional and spiritual states of stress and can immediately start to strengthen self-identity. Deep Immune will help to strengthen the immune system on a number of levels.

Exposure to novel pathogenic organisms through travel to foreign countries, visits to the sick, mixing with groups at conferences, returning to school, and the like can be challenging. Mental and emotional preparedness combined with a week or two of Deep Immune before the event is good prevention.

I cannot over-emphasize the importance of inner self-awareness and emotional, mental, and spiritual preparedness in dealing with stressful situations.

When to Avoid Herbal Remedies

Generally speaking, appropriate herbal remedies can be used safely and with benefit at virtually any time and under any circumstance. However, the differences between individuals and their specific circumstances can make the decision when to use herbal remedies difficult to discern.

The main reason to avoid herbal remedies are:

- if you are afraid of them, don't believe you need them, don't want them, are tired of taking them, or believe they are harming you.
- if you do not know what you are doing and do not have the skilled help of a knowledgeable, suitably trained person that you trust.

- if you feel that herbal medicine cannot be blended in a beneficial way with other medical disciplines upon which you are relying for your survival or recovery from illness.

Confusion often arises because people may equate herbal remedies with drugs. While they can and do have drug-like effects, most herbs are not like drugs in any way. They are nourishing, balancing, supporting, and healing to every cell, tissue, and organ of the body and also to the emotions, mind, and spirit. This means that a knowledgeable person can draw on the healing power of herbs at any or all times to assist and teach him on the journey of healing.

IN CONCLUSION

Herbs are our allies on the journey of healing that is life, and herbs can help us in every circumstance. To develop the most mutually beneficial relationship with healing plants, we must come to know them as fellow creatures through all our faculties—vision, touch, taste, and smell, emotions, intellect and feelings—but especially in our hearts.

BIBLIOGRAPHY

Bach, Edward. *The Twelve Healers and Other Remedies*. Essex, England: C.W. Daniel Co. Ltd., 1933.

Hay, Louise, L. *You Can Heal Your Life*. Hay House Inc., 1987.

Hobbs, Christopher. *Medicinal Mushrooms*. Santa Cruz, CA: Botanica Press, 1987

Hoffman, David. *Medical Herbalism: The Science and Practice of Herbal Medicine*. Rochester, VT: Healing Arts Press, 2003.

Holmes, Peter. *Jade Remedies: A Chinese Herbal Reference for the West* (2 vols., 1st ed.). Boulder, CO: Snow Lotus Press, 1996.

Kirchfeld, Friedhelm and Boyle, Wade. *Nature Doctors: Pioneers in Naturopathic Medicine*. Portland, OR: Medicina Biologica, and East Palestine, OH: Buckeye Naturopathic Press, reprint in 2000 of 1994 edition.

Malin, Shimon. *Nature Loves to Hide: Quantum Physics and the Nature of Reality, a Western Perspective.* NY: Oxford University Press, 2001.

Pert, Candace B., Ph.D. *Molecules of Emotion.* New York, NY: Scribners, 1997.

Scudder, John M., M.D. *Specific Medication.* (Reprint of 15th ed., 1903) Portland, OR: Eclectic Medical Publications, 1985.

Teeguarden, Ron. *Chinese Tonic Herbs.* Tokyo and New York: Japan Publications Inc., 1985.

Teeguarden, Ron. *Radiant Health: The Ancient Wisdom of the Chinese Tonic Herbs.* New York: Warner Books, 1998.

Weeks, Nora. *The Medical Discoveries of Edward Bach Physician.* Essex, England: C.W. Daniel Co. Ltd., 1973.